POCKET COMPANION FOR

Physical Examination
& Health Assessment

CAROLYN JARVIS, PhD, APRN, CNP

Professor of Nursing
Illinois Wesleyan University
Bloomington, Illinois
and
Family Nurse Practitioner
Bloomington, Illinois

With Ann Eckhardt, PhD, RN

Associate Professor of Nursing
Illinois Wesleyan University
Bloomington, Illinois

8TH EDITION

ELSEVIER

Original Illustrations by
Pat Thomas, CMI, FAMI
East Troy, Wisconsin

POCKET COMPANION FOR PHYSICAL EXAMINATION
AND HEALTH ASSESSMENT, EIGHTH EDITION

ISBN: 978-0-323-53202-0

Notice

Practitioners and researchers must always rely on their own experience and knowledge in evaluating and using any information, methods, compounds or experiments described herein. Because of rapid advances in the medical sciences, in particular, independent verification of diagnoses and drug dosages should be made. To the fullest extent of the law, no responsibility is assumed by Elsevier, authors, editors or contributors for any injury and/or damage to persons or property as a matter of products liability, negligence or otherwise, or from any use or operation of any methods, products, instructions, or ideas contained in the material herein.

Previous editions copyrighted 2016, 2012, 2008, 2004, 2000, 1996, 1993.

International Standard Book Number: 978-0-323-53202-0

Executive Content Strategist: Lee Henderson
Senior Content Development Specialist: Heather Bays
Publishing Services Manager: Julie Eddy
Senior Project Manager: Jodi M. Willard
Design Direction: Brian Salisbury

Printed in the United States of America

Last digit is the print number: 9   8   7   6   5   4   3   2

ELSEVIER

3251 Riverport Lane
St. Louis,
Missouri
63043

  Working together to grow libraries in developing countries

www.elsevier.com • www.bookaid.org

The eighth edition of *Pocket Companion for Physical Examination and Health Assessment* is designed for two groups—those who need a practical clinical reference and those acquiring beginning assessment skills.

First, the *Pocket Companion* is intended as an adjunct to Jarvis' *Physical Examination and Health Assessment*, 8th edition. The *Pocket Companion* is a memory prompt for those who have studied physical assessment and wish to have a reminder when in the clinic. The *Pocket Companion* has all the essentials—health history points, exam steps for each body system, normal versus abnormal findings, heart sounds, lung sounds, neurologic checks. *The Pocket Companion* is useful when you forget a step in the exam sequence, when you wish to be sure your assessment is complete, when you need to review the findings that are normal versus abnormal, or when you are faced with an unfamiliar technique or a new clinical area. Its portable size and binding make it perfect for a lab coat pocket or home health bag.

Second, the *Pocket Companion*, 8th edition, is an independent primer of basic assessment skills. It is well suited to programs that integrate an assessment course covering well people of all ages into other arching courses. The *Pocket Companion* has the complete steps to perform a health history and physical examination on a well person. It includes pertinent developmental content for pediatric, pregnant, and aging adult patients. Although the description of each exam step is stated concisely, there is enough information given to study and learn exam techniques. However, because there is no room in the *Pocket Companion* for theories, principles, or detailed explanations, students using the *Pocket Companion* as a beginning text must have a thorough didactic presentation of assessment methods as well as tutored practice.

The *Pocket Companion*, 8th edition, is revised and updated to match the revision of the parent text, *Physical Examination and Health Assessment*, 8th edition, including many new examination photos, abnormal findings photos, and full-color art. Numerous tables of Abnormal Findings are also new to the 8th edition, including Delirium, Dementia, and Depression.

An updated section on the **Electronic Health Record** has been integrated into Chapter 21, Bedside Assessment and Electronic Documentation. This section outlines charting, and narrative recording provides examples of how to document assessment findings.

For those times when readers need detailed coverage of a particular technique or finding, it is easily found through numerous cross-references to pages in *Physical Examination and Health Assessment*, 8th edition.

As you thumb through the *Pocket Companion,* note these features:
- Health history and exam steps are concise yet complete.
- Method of examination is clear, orderly, and easy to follow.
- Abnormal findings are described briefly in a column adjacent to the normal range of findings.
- Sample charting is now included in all applicable chapters, illustrating the documentation of findings.
- A key point is described for Health Promotion and Patient Teaching in each chapter.
- Tables are presented at the end of chapters to fully illustrate important information.
- Selected Cultural Competence information highlights this important aspect of a health assessment.

- Developmental Competence content includes age-specific information for pediatric, pregnant, and older adult groups.
- Summary checklists for each chapter form a cue card of exam steps to remember.
- Integration of the complete health assessment is presented in Chapter 20.
- Selected artwork from *Physical Examination and Health Assessment*, 8th edition, illustrates the pertinent anatomy.

Acknowledgments

I am grateful to those on the team at Elsevier who worked on the *Pocket Companion*. My thanks extend to Lee Henderson, Executive Content Strategist; Heather Bays, Senior Content Development Specialist; Jodi Willard, Senior Project Manager; Julie Eddy, Publishing Services Manager; and Brian Salisbury, Design, for their patient and attentive monitoring of every step in the production of the *Pocket Companion*.

Thank you also to Leslie Foster, Illustrator/Designer, who hand-dummied every page and crafted each page layout for clarity and alignment. Finally, I am very grateful and delighted to welcome my colleague Ann Eckhardt, PhD, RN, to the 8th edition. Dr. Eckhardt revised Chapters 1, 2, 3, 4, and Chapters 20 and 21. Welcome aboard!

Carolyn Jarvis

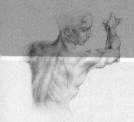

CHAPTER 1

The Interview and Complete Health History

The health history is important in beginning to identify the person's health strengths and problems and as a bridge to the next step in data collection, the physical examination.

The health history collects **subjective data**, what the person says about himself or herself. This is the first and best chance that a person has to tell you what *he* or *she* perceives his or her health state to be.

EXTERNAL FACTORS

Ensure Privacy. Aim for geographic privacy—a private room. If geographic privacy is not available, "psychological privacy" afforded by curtained partitions may suffice as long as the person feels sure that no one can overhear the conversation or interrupt.

Refuse Interruptions. You need this time to concentrate and establish rapport.

Physical Environment

- Set the room temperature at a comfortable level.
- Provide sufficient lighting.
- Reduce noise.
- Remove distracting objects.
- Maintain the distance between you and the patient at 4 to 5 feet (twice an arm's length).
- Arrange equal-status seating. Both of you should be comfortably seated at eye level. Avoid sitting behind a desk or bedside table placed so it looks like a barrier.
- Avoid standing.

There are three phases to each interview: an introduction, a working phase, and a termination (or closing).

INTRODUCING THE INTERVIEW

Address the patient using his or her surname. Introduce yourself and state your role in the agency (if you are a student, say so). If you are gathering a complete history, give the reason for this interview.

THE WORKING PHASE

The working phase is the data-gathering phase. It involves your questions to the patient and your responses to what he or she has said. There are two types of questions: open-ended and closed (or direct). Each type has a different place and function in the interview.

Open-Ended Questions

An open-ended question asks for narrative information. It states the topic to be discussed, but only in general terms. Use it to begin the interview, to introduce a new section of questions, and whenever the person introduces a new topic. Examples are, "Tell me what brings you in today" and "What brings you to the hospital?"

Closed or Direct Questions

Closed or direct questions ask for specific information. They elicit a one- or two-word answer, a "yes" or "no," or a forced choice. Use direct questions after the person's narrative to fill in any details that he or she may have omitted. Also use direct questions when you need many specific facts such as when asking about past health problems or during the review of systems.

Responses

As the person talks, your role is to encourage free expression but not let him or her wander. The following responses help you gather data without cutting off the person.

Facilitation. Your facilitative response encourages the patient to say more, to continue with the story, e.g., "mm-hmm," "go on," "continue," "uh-huh," or simply by nodding.

Silence. Your silence communicates that the patient has time to think and organize what he or she wishes to say without interruption from you. Silence also gives you a chance to observe the person unobtrusively and to note nonverbal cues.

Reflection. A reflective response echoes the patient's own words. Reflection involves repeating part of what the person has just said. It focuses further attention on a specific phrase and helps the person continue in his or her own way.

Empathy. An empathic response recognizes a feeling and puts it into words. It names the feeling and allows its expression. When you use an empathic response, the patient feels accepted and can deal with the feeling openly. Empathic responses include saying, "This must be very hard for you" or just placing your hand on the person's arm.

Clarification. Use the clarification response when the patient's word choice is ambiguous or confusing, e.g., "Tell me what you mean by 'tired blood.'"

Confrontation. In this case you have observed a certain action, feeling, or statement; you now focus the person's attention on it. This can focus on a discrepancy: "You say it doesn't hurt, but when I touch you here, you grimace." It can also focus on the patient's affect: "You look sad" or "You sound angry."

Interpretation. An interpretive response is based not on direct observation (as is confrontation) but on your inference or conclusion. Interpretation links events, makes associations, or implies cause: "It seems that every time you feel the stomach pain, you have had some kind of stress in your life."

Explanation. With these statements you share factual and objective information. This may be for orientation to the agency setting: "Your dinner comes at 5:30 PM"; or it may be to explain cause: "The reason you cannot eat or drink before your blood test is that the food will change the test results."

Summary. This is a final review of what you understand the patient has said. It condenses the facts and presents a survey of how you perceive the patient's health problem or need. It also allows the patient to correct misperceptions.

CLOSING THE INTERVIEW

The meeting should end gracefully. To ease into the closing, ask the patient, "Is there anything else you would like to mention?" Give the person a final opportunity for self-expression. Then give a summary or recapitulation of what you have learned during the interview. This is a final statement of what you and the patient agree his or her health state to be.

TEN TRAPS OF INTERVIEWING

Nonproductive, defeating verbal messages restrict the patient's response. They are obstacles to obtaining complete data and establishing rapport.

1. Providing False Reassurance. Such statements as "Now don't worry, I'm sure you'll be all right" are courage builders that relieve *your* anxiety and give you a false sense of having provided comfort. However, for the patient these statements close off communication. They trivialize anxiety and effectively deny further discussion.

2. Giving Unwanted Advice. A person describes a problem to you, ending with "What would you do?" If you answer, "If I were you, I'd …," you have shifted the accountability for decision making from the patient to you. The person has not worked out his or her own solution and has learned nothing about himself or herself.

3. Using Authority. "Your doctor/ nurse knows best" is a response that promotes dependency and inferiority.

4. Using Avoidance Language. People use euphemisms such as "passed on" to avoid reality or to hide their feelings.

5. Engaging in Distancing. Distancing is the use of impersonal speech to put space between a threat and oneself, e.g., "There is a lump in *the* left breast."

6. Using Professional Jargon. Use of jargon sounds exclusionary and paternalistic. You need to adjust your vocabulary to the patient but should avoid sounding condescending.

7. Using Leading or Biased Questions. Asking such questions as "You don't smoke, do you?" implies that one answer is "better" than another.

8. Talking Too Much. Some examiners associate helpfulness with how much they talk. They think they have met the patient's needs. Just the opposite is true.

9. Interrupting. When you think you know what patients will say, you interrupt and cut them off.

10. Using "Why" Questions. The adult's use of "why" questions usually implies blame and condemnation and puts the patient on the defensive.

Nonverbal Skills

Nonverbal messages that are productive and enhancing to the relationship are those that show attentiveness and unconditional acceptance. Defeating and nonproductive nonverbal behaviors are those of inattentiveness, authority, and superiority (Table 1.1).

TABLE 1.1	Nonverbal Behaviors of the Interviewer
Positive	**Negative**
Appropriate professional appearance	Appearance objectionable to patient
Equal-status seating	Standing
Close placement to patient	Sitting behind desk, far away, turned away
Relaxed open posture	Tense posture
Leaning slightly toward person	Slouched back posture
Occasional facilitation gestures	Critical or distracting gestures: pointing finger, clenched fist, finger-tapping, foot-swinging, looking at watch
Facial animation, interest	Bland expression, yawning, tight mouth
Appropriate smiling	Frowning, lip biting
Appropriate eye contact	Shifting eyes, avoiding eye contact, focusing on notes
Moderate tone of voice	Strident, high-pitched tone
Moderate rate of speech	Rate too slow or too fast
Appropriate touch	Too frequent or inappropriate touch

THE HEALTH HISTORY: THE ADULT

Biographic Data

This information includes name; address; telephone number; age; birth date; birthplace; sex; relationship status; race; ethnic origin; and occupation, usual and present.

Source of History

The history may be provided by the patient or a surrogate.

Reason for Seeking Care

This is a brief, spontaneous statement in the patient's own words that describes the reason for the visit.

Present Health or History of Present Illness

This is a chronologic record of the reason for seeking care, from the time of the onset of the symptoms until now. Start when the person first noticed the symptoms and work forward to the present. Your final summary of any symptom the patient has should include these *critical characteristics*, organized into the mnemonic PQRSTU to help remember all the points.

P. Provocative or **palliative**. What brings it on? What were you doing when you first noticed it? What makes it better? Worse?

Q. Quality or **quantity**. How does it look, feel, sound? How intense/severe is it?

R. Region or **radiation**. Where is it? Does it spread anywhere?

S. Severity scale. How bad is it (on a scale ranging from 1 to 10)? Is it getting better, worse, staying the same?

T. Timing. Onset—Exactly when did it first occur? Duration—How long did it last? Frequency—How often does it occur?

U. Understand *patient's perception* of the problem. What do you think it means?

Past Health

Childhood Illnesses. Measles, mumps, rubella, chickenpox, pertussis, strep throat, rheumatic fever, scarlet fever, and poliomyelitis.

Accidents or Injuries. Head injuries, auto accidents, fractures.

Serious or Chronic Illnesses. Diabetes, hypertension, heart disease, sickle-cell anemia, cancer, and seizure disorder.

Hospitalizations and Operations. Name of surgery, hospital, date.

Obstetric History. The number of pregnancies (gravidity), number of deliveries in which the fetus reached viability (parity), number of incomplete pregnancies or abortions, and number of living children. This is recorded as G_P_Ab_Liv_ (e.g., G3 P2 Ab1 Liv 2).

Immunizations. All immunizations (measles/mumps/rubella, poliomyelitis, diphtheria/pertussis/tetanus, hepatitis B, hepatitis A in selected areas, *Haemophilus influenzae* type b, and pneumococcal vaccine). Also note the last tetanus immunization, last tuberculosis skin test, and last flu shot.

Last Examination Date. The most recent physical, dental, vision, hearing, electrocardiogram, and chest x-ray examinations.

Allergies. Medication, food, environmental agent. Note reaction.

Current Medications. All prescription and over-the-counter medications, including laxatives, vitamins, birth control pills, aspirin, and antacids.

Family History

The age and health or the age and cause of death of blood relatives such as parents, grandparents, and siblings. The age and health of spouse and children. Specifically any family history of heart disease, high blood pressure, stroke, diabetes, blood disorders, cancer, sickle-cell anemia, arthritis, allergies, obesity, alcoholism, mental illness, seizure disorder, kidney disease, or tuberculosis. Construct a family tree, or genogram, to show this information clearly and concisely (Fig. 1.1).

Review of Systems

General Overall Health State. Present weight (gain or loss, period of

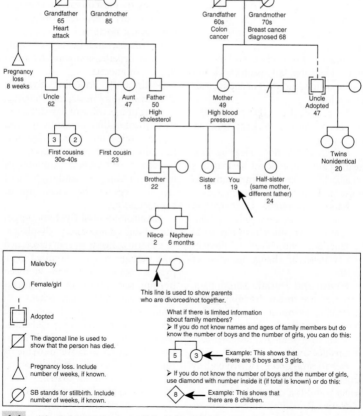

1.1 A family tree, or genogram. (Adapted from the American Society of Human Genetics, www.ashg.org, 2004.)

time, by diet or other factors), fatigue, weakness or malaise, fever, chills, and sweats or night sweats.

Skin. History of skin disease (eczema, psoriasis, hives), pigment or color change, change in mole, excessive dryness or moisture, pruritus, excessive bruising, and rash or lesion.

Health Promotion. Amount of sun exposure.

Hair. Recent loss, change in texture.

Nails. Change in shape, color, or brittleness.

Head. Unusually frequent or severe headache, any head injury, dizziness (syncope), or vertigo.

Eyes. Difficulty with vision (decreased acuity, blurring, blind spots), eye pain, diplopia (double vision), redness or swelling, watering or discharge, and glaucoma or cataracts.

Health Promotion. Glasses or contact lens use, last vision check and glaucoma test, and ways of coping with vision loss.

Ears. Earaches, infections, discharge and its characteristics, tinnitus, or vertigo.

Health Promotion. Hearing loss, hearing aid use, effect of hearing loss on daily life, exposure to environmental noise, and method of cleaning ears.

Nose and Sinuses. Discharge and its characteristics, unusually frequent or severe colds, any sinus pain, nasal obstruction, nosebleeds, allergies or hay fever, or change in sense of smell.

Mouth and Throat. Mouth pain, frequent sore throat, bleeding gums, toothache, lesion in mouth or on tongue, dysphagia, hoarseness or voice change, or altered taste. History of tonsillectomy.

Health Promotion. Pattern of daily dental care, use of prosthesis (dentures, bridge), and last dental checkup.

Neck. Pain, limitation of motion, lumps or swelling, enlarged or tender nodes, or goiter.

Breast. Pain, lump, nipple discharge, rash, or breast disease.

Health Promotion. Breast self-examination method and frequency; last mammogram.

Axilla. Tenderness, lump or swelling, rash.

Respiratory System. History of lung diseases (asthma, emphysema, bronchitis, pneumonia, tuberculosis); chest pain with breathing; wheezing or noisy breathing; shortness of breath; how much activity produces shortness of breath; cough; sputum (color, amount); hemoptysis; and toxin or pollution exposure.

Cardiovascular System. Precordial or retrosternal pain; palpitation; cyanosis; dyspnea on exertion (specify amount of exertion); orthopnea; paroxysmal nocturnal dyspnea; nocturia; edema; and history of heart murmur, hypertension, coronary artery disease, or anemia.

Peripheral Vascular System. Coldness, numbness and tingling, swelling of legs (time of day and activity), discoloration in hands or feet, varicose veins, intermittent claudication, thrombophlebitis, or ulcers.

Health Promotion. Amount of long-term sitting or standing, habit of crossing legs at the knees, use of support hose.

Gastrointestinal System. Appetite; food intolerance; dysphagia; heartburn; indigestion; pain (associated with eating); other abdominal pain; pyrosis (esophageal and stomach burning sensation with sour eructation); nausea and vomiting (character); vomiting blood; history of abdominal disease (ulcer, liver, or gallbladder; jaundice; appendicitis; colitis); flatulence; frequency of bowel movements (any recent change); stool characteristics; constipation or diarrhea; black stools; rectal bleeding; or rectal conditions (hemorrhoids, fistula).

Health Promotion. Last serum cholesterol test, stool occult blood.

Urinary System. Frequency or urgency; nocturia (recent change), dysuria, polyuria, or oliguria; hesitancy or straining; narrowed stream; urine color (cloudy or presence of blood), incontinence; history of urinary disease (kidney disease, kidney stones, urinary tract infections, prostate disease); or pain in flank, groin, suprapubic region, or low back.

Health Promotion. Use of Kegel exercises; measures to avoid or treat urinary tract infections.

Male Genital System. Penile or testicular pain, sores or lesions, penile discharge, lumps, or hernia.

Health Promotion. Testicular self-examination method and frequency.

Female Genital System. Menstrual history (age at menarche, last menstrual period, cycle and duration, amenorrhea or menorrhagia, premenstrual pain or dysmenorrhea, intermenstrual spotting), vaginal itching, discharge and its characteristics, age at menopause, menopausal signs or symptoms, or postmenopausal bleeding.

Health Promotion. Last gynecologic checkup, last Pap test.

Sexual Health. Current sexual activity, level of sexual satisfaction of patient and partner, dyspareunia (for female); changes in erection or ejaculation (for male); use of contraceptive and satisfaction with it; any known or suspected contact with a partner who has a sexually transmitted infection (gonorrhea, herpes, chlamydia, venereal warts, HIV/AIDS, or syphilis).

Musculoskeletal System. History of arthritis or gout. Joint pain, stiffness, swelling (location, migratory nature), deformity, limitation of motion, or noise with joint motion. Muscle pain, cramps, weakness, gait problems, or problems with coordinated activities. Other pain (location and radiation to extremities), stiffness, limitation of motion, or history of back pain or disc disease.

Health Promotion. Distance walked per day; effect of limited range of motion on daily activities such as grooming, feeding, toileting, or dressing; and use of mobility aids.

Neurologic System. History of seizure disorder, stroke, fainting, or blackouts. Motor function: any weakness, tic or tremor, paralysis, or coordination problems. Sensory function: any numbness and tingling (paresthesia). Cognitive function: any memory disorder (recent or distant, disorientation). Mental status: nervousness, mood change, depression, or history of mental health dysfunction or hallucinations.

Hematologic System. Bleeding of skin or mucous membranes, excessive bruising, lymph node swelling, exposure to toxic agents or radiation, or blood transfusion and reactions.

Endocrine System. History of diabetes or diabetic symptoms (polyuria, polydipsia, polyphagia). History of thyroid disease, intolerance to heat and cold, change in skin pigmentation or texture, excessive sweating. Relationship between appetite and weight, abnormal hair distribution, nervousness, tremors, or need for hormone therapy.

Functional Assessment (Activities of Daily Living)

Functional assessment measures a person's self-care ability in the areas of physical health; activities of daily living (ADLs) such as bathing, dressing, toileting, and eating; instrumental activities of daily living (IADLs), which are those needed for independent living such as housekeeping, shopping, and cooking; nutritional status; social relationships and resources; self-concept and coping; and home environment. These questions provide data on the lifestyle and type of living environment to which the person is accustomed.

Self-Esteem/Self-Concept. Education (last grade completed, other significant training); financial status (income adequate for lifestyle and/or health concerns); and values and belief system (religious practices and perception of personal strengths).

Activity/Exercise. A daily profile reflecting usual daily activities. Ability to perform ADLs—independent or needs assistance. Ability to tolerate activity or use prostheses or mobility aids. Leisure activities enjoyed and exercise pattern (type, amount per day or week, warm-up session, response of body to exercise).

Sleep/Rest. Sleep patterns, any sleep aids, or daytime naps.

Nutrition/Elimination. All food and beverages consumed during the past 24 hours: "Is that menu typical?" Eating habits and current appetite. "Who buys and prepares food? Are finances adequate for food? Who is present at mealtimes?" Any food allergy or intolerance; daily intake of caffeine (coffee, tea, cola drinks).

Interpersonal Relationships/Resources. Social roles: "What's your role in your family? How would you say you get along with family, friends, and co-workers?" Support systems composed of family and significant others: "To whom could you go for support with a problem at work, with your health, or with a personal problem?" Amount of time spent alone: "Is it pleasurable or isolating?"

Coping and Stress Management. Stresses in life now and in the past year, any change in lifestyle or any current stress, and any steps taken to relieve stress.

Personal Habits. Alcohol: "When was your last drink of alcohol? How much did you drink that time? Have you ever had a drinking problem?" Smoking: "Do you smoke? At what age did you start? How many packs do you smoke per day? How many years have you smoked?" Street drugs: "Have you ever tried any drugs such as marijuana, cocaine, amphetamines, or barbiturates? How often do you use these drugs? How has usage affected your work or social relationships?"

Environment/Hazards. Housing and neighborhood (live alone, know neighbors, safety of area, adequate heat and utilities, access to transportation, involved in community services) and environmental health (hazards in workplace, hazards at home, use of seatbelts, geographic or occupational exposures, travel or residence in other countries).

Intimate Partner Violence. "How are things at home? Do you feel safe?" If the person responds to feeling unsafe, follow up with "Have you ever been emotionally or physically abused by your partner or someone important to you? Within the last year have you been hit, slapped, kicked, pushed, shoved, or otherwise physically hurt by your partner or ex-partner? If yes, by whom? Number of times? Does your partner ever force you to have sex? Are you afraid of your partner or ex-partner?"

Occupational Health. "Please describe your job. Ever worked with any health hazard, asbestos, inhalants, chemicals, repetitive motion? Wear or use any protective equipment? Any work programs to monitor your exposure? Any health problems now that you think are related to work? What do you like or dislike about your work?"

Perception of Health

"How do you define health? How do you view your situation now? What are your concerns? What do you think will happen in the future? What are your health goals? What do you expect from us as nurses, physicians, other health care providers?"

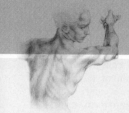

CHAPTER 2

Mental Status Assessment

Mental status is a person's emotional and cognitive functioning. Optimal functioning aims toward simultaneous life satisfaction in work, in caring relationships, and within the self.

Mental status cannot be scrutinized directly like the characteristics of skin or heart sounds. Its functioning is *inferred* through assessment of an individual's behaviors:

Consciousness: Awareness of one's own existence, feelings, and thoughts and of the environment

Language: Using the voice to communicate one's thoughts and feelings

Mood and affect: Both of these elements deal with prevailing feelings; mood is a prolonged display of feelings that colors the whole emotional life, whereas affect is a temporary expression of feelings

Orientation: Awareness of the objective world in relation to the self

Attention: The power of concentration; the ability to focus on one specific thing without being distracted

Memory: The ability to note and store experiences and perceptions for later recall; *recent* memory evokes day-to-day events, and *remote* memory brings up many years of experiences

Abstract reasoning: Pondering of a deeper meaning beyond the concrete and literal

Thought process: The *way* a person thinks; the logical train of thought

Thought content: *What* a person thinks; specific ideas, beliefs, and use of words

Perceptions: Awareness of objects through any of the five senses

THE MENTAL STATUS EXAMINATION

The full mental status examination is a systematic check of emotional and cognitive functioning. However, the steps described here rarely need to be taken in their entirety. Usually you can assess mental status through the context of the health history interview. During that time keep in mind the four main headings of mental status assessment:

Appearance
Behavior
Cognition
Thought processes

or **A, B, C, T.**

In every mental status examination note these factors from the health history that could affect your interpretation of findings:
- Any known illnesses or health problems such as alcohol disorders or chronic renal disease
- Current medications with side effects causing confusion or depression
- The educational level and usual behavior; note this as the normal baseline and do not expect

performance on the mental status examination to exceed it

- Responses to personal history questions, indicating current stress, social interaction patterns, sleep habits, drug and alcohol use

Appearance

Posture and Position. Posture is erect, and position is relaxed.

Body Movements. Voluntary, deliberate, coordinated, and smooth and even.

Dress. Appropriate for setting, season, age, gender, and social group. Clothing fits and is put on appropriately.

Grooming and Hygiene. The person is clean and well groomed; hair is neat and clean; women have moderate or no make-up; men are clean shaven, or the beard or mustache is well groomed. Nails are clean (although some jobs leave nails chronically dirty). Note that a disheveled appearance in a previously well-groomed person is significant. Use care in interpreting clothing that is disheveled, bizarre, or in poor repair because this sometimes reflects the person's economic status or a deliberate fashion trend.

Pupils. Note pupil size and reaction to light.

Behavior

Level of Consciousness. The person is alert, aware of stimuli from the environment and within the self, and responds appropriately (Table 2.1, p. 13).

Facial Expression. The look is appropriate to the situation and changes appropriately with the topic. There is comfortable eye contact unless precluded by cultural norm.

Speech. *Quality:* The person makes laryngeal sounds effortlessly and shares conversation appropriately.

The *pace* of the conversation is moderate, and stream of talking is fluent.

Articulation (ability to form words) is clear and understandable.

Word choice is effortless and appropriate to educational level. The person completes sentences, occasionally pausing to think.

Mood/Affect. Determine this by body language and facial expression and by asking, "How do you feel today?" or "How do you usually feel?" The mood should be appropriate to the person's place and condition and should change appropriately with topics. The person is willing to cooperate with you.

Cognitive Functions

Orientation. You can discern orientation through the course of the interview. Assess:

Time: Day of week, date, year, season
Place: Where person lives, present location, type of building, name of city and state
Person: Own name, age, who examiner is

Many hospitalized people normally have trouble with the exact date but are fully oriented to other items.

Attention Span. Check the person's ability to concentrate by noting whether he or she completes a thought without wandering. Note any distractibility or difficulty attending to you or give a series of directions to follow and note the correct sequence of behaviors. Be aware that attention span commonly is impaired in people who are anxious, fatigued, or drug intoxicated.

Recent Memory. Assess recent memory in the context of the interview by the 24-hour diet recall.

Remote Memory. In the context of the interview, ask the person verifiable past events, e.g., past health, first job, birthday and anniversary dates, and historic events.

Judgment. To assess judgment in the context of the interview, note what the person says about job plans, social or family obligations, and plans for the future. Also ask the person to describe the rationale for personal health care and how he or she has decided about complying with prescribed health regimens. The person's actions and decisions should be realistic.

Thought Processes and Perceptions

Thought Processes. Ask yourself whether the patient makes sense and whether you can follow what he or she is saying. The way a person thinks should be logical, goal directed, coherent, and relevant. The person should complete a thought.

Thought Content. *What* the person says should be consistent and logical.

Perceptions. The person should be consistently aware of reality. His or her perceptions should be congruent with yours. Ask the following questions:
- "How do people treat you?"
- "Do other people talk about you?"
- "Do you feel as if you are being watched, followed, or controlled?"
- "Is your imagination very active?"
- "Have you heard your name when alone?"

Screen for Anxiety Disorders. Anxiety and depression are the two most common mental health problems seen in people seeking general medical care. Anxiety disorders are common, disabling, and often untreated. However, you can screen for core anxiety symptoms by asking the first two questions from the seven-item generalized anxiety disorder (GAD) scale (Kroenke et al., 2007). *Over the last 2 weeks, how often have you been bothered by the following problems? (1) Feeling nervous, anxious, or on edge;* *and (2) Not being able to stop or control worrying.*

NOT AT ALL	SEVERAL DAYS	MORE THAN HALF THE DAYS	NEARLY EVERY DAY
0	1	2	3

Scores on this GAD subscale range from 0 to 6; a score of 0 suggests that no anxiety disorder is present, while a score ≥ 3 indicates anxiety. If the score is ≥ 3, a full assessment for anxiety should be completed.

Screen for Depression. Many formal screening tools are available. However, a shorter method, asking two simple questions about depressed mood and anhedonia, detects a majority of depressed patients (Lakkis & Mahmassani, 2015).

Thus you can ask: *Over the past 2 weeks, how often have you been bothered by any of the following problems? (1) Feeling little interest or pleasure in doing things, and (2) Feeling down, depressed, or hopeless.*

NOT AT ALL	SEVERAL DAYS	MORE THAN HALF THE DAYS	NEARLY EVERY DAY
0	1	2	3

If the person answers *several days or more,* administer the full PHQ-9 (see Jarvis: *Physical Examination and Health Assessment,* 8th ed., p. 69).

Screen for Suicidal Thoughts. When the person expresses feelings of sadness, hopelessness, or despair or grief, it is important to assess any possible risk of physical self-harm. Begin with more general questions. If you receive affirmative answers, continue with more specific questions:
- "Have you ever thought of hurting yourself?"
- "Do you feel like hurting yourself now?"
- "Do you have a plan to hurt yourself?"

- "How would you do it?"
- "What would happen if you were dead?"
- "How would other people react if you were dead?"
- Who could you tell if you felt like killing yourself?

Do not skip these questions if you have the slightest hint that they are appropriate. You may be the only health professional to pick up clues to suicide risk. You are responsible for encouraging the person to talk about suicidal thoughts. You cannot always prevent a suicide when someone really wishes to kill himself or herself. However, most people are ambivalent, and you can buy time and help the person find an alternate solution to the situation.

COGNITIVE FUNCTION

The Mini-Mental State Examination (MMSE) and Montreal Cognitive Assessment (MoCA) are short cognitive assessment tools that can be used to screen for dementia and cognitive impairment. The MoCA is more sensitive to mild cognitive impairment than the MMSE. Both screening tools require only pencil and paper and can be administered in less than 10 minutes.

For more information on abnormalities of mood and affect, delirium and dementia, substance use disorders, mood disorders, and anxiety disorders, see Table 2.2 and Jarvis: *Physical Examination and Health Assessment,* 8th ed., pp. 70-71.

DOCUMENTATION

Sample Charting

Appearance: Person's posture is erect, with no involuntary body movements. Dress and grooming are appropriate for season and setting.

Behavior: Person is alert, with appropriate facial expression and fluent, understandable speech. Affect and verbal responses are appropriate.

Cognitive functions: Oriented to time, person, place. Able to attend cooperatively with examiner. Recent and remote memory intact. Can recall four unrelated words at 5-, 10-, and 30-minute testing intervals. Future plans include returning home and to local university once individual therapy is established and medication is adjusted.

Thought processes: Perceptions and thought processes are logical and coherent. No suicide ideation.

Score on Mini-Mental State Examination is 28.

ABNORMAL FINDINGS

TABLE 2.1	Levels of Consciousness

The terms below are commonly used in clinical practice. They spread over a continuum from full alertness to deep coma. They are qualitative and therefore are not always reliable. (A quantitative tool that serves the same purpose and eliminates ambiguity is the Glasgow Coma Scale [see Chapter 16].) However, these terms are widely accepted and are useful as long as all co-workers agree on definitions and are consistent in their application.

To increase clarity when using these terms, also record:

1. The level of stimulus used, ranging progressively from:
   a. Name called in normal tone of voice
   b. Name called in loud voice
   c. Light touch on person's arm
   d. Vigorous shake of shoulder
   e. Pain applied
2. The person's response
   a. Amount and quality of movement
   b. Presence and coherence of speech
   c. Opens eyes and makes eye contact
3. What the person does on cessation of your stimulus
   (1) **Alert**
       Awake or readily aroused, oriented, fully aware of external and internal stimuli, and responds appropriately; conducts meaningful interpersonal interactions
   (2) **Lethargic (or Somnolent)**
       Not fully alert, drifts off to sleep when not stimulated, can be aroused to name when called in normal voice but looks drowsy; responds appropriately to questions or commands, but thinking seems slow and fuzzy; inattentive, loses train of thought; spontaneous movements decreased
   (3) **Obtunded**
       (Transitional state between lethargy and stupor; some sources omit this level.) Sleeps most of time, difficult to arouse (needs loud shout or vigorous shake), acts confused when aroused; converses in monosyllables, speech may be mumbled and incoherent; requires constant stimulation for even marginal cooperation
   (4) **Stupor or Semi-Coma**
       Spontaneously unconscious, responds only to vigorous shake or pain, has appropriate motor response (i.e., withdraws hand to avoid pain); otherwise can only groan, mumble, or move restlessly but retains reflex activity
   (5) **Coma**
       Completely unconscious, makes no response to pain or to any external or internal stimuli (e.g., when suctioned, will not try to push the catheter away); light coma has some reflex activity but no purposeful movement; deep coma has no motor response

Acute Confusional State (Delirium)

Has clouding of consciousness (dulled cognition, impaired alertness), is inattentive, makes incoherent conversation, has impaired recent memory, and is confabulatory for recent events; is often agitated and has visual hallucinations; is disoriented, with confusion worse at night when environmental stimuli are decreased

Modified from Strub, R. L., & Black, F. W. (2000). *The mental status examination in neurology* (4th ed.). Philadelphia: F.A. Davis.

TABLE 2.2	Delirium, Dementia, and Depression

Delirium is an acute confusional state, potentially preventable in hospitalized persons. Characterized by disorientation, disordered thinking and perceptions (illusions and hallucinations), defective memory, agitation, inattention.

Dementia is a chronic progressive loss of cognitive and intellectual functions, although perception and consciousness are intact. Characterized by disorientation, impaired judgment, memory loss.

Depression is a long-term depressed mood (≥ previous 2 weeks), with lack of pleasure; disturbed sleep and appetite; feelings of hopelessness, guilt, worthlessness, sadness, loneliness and despair; suicide ideation.

See the following comparisons.

	Delirium	Dementia	Depression
Onset	Sudden, over hours to days	Slowly, over months	May have been gradual, with exacerbation during crisis or stress
Cause or contributing factors	Hypoglycemia, fever, dehydration, hypotension; infection, other conditions that disrupt body homeostasis; adverse drug reaction; head injury; change in environment (e.g., hospitalization); pain; emotional stress; substance abuse	Alzheimer disease, vascular disease, human immunodeficiency virus infection, neurologic disease, chronic alcoholism, head trauma	Lifelong history, losses, loneliness, crises, declining health, medical conditions
Cognition	Impaired memory, judgment, calculations, attention span; can fluctuate through the day	Impaired memory, judgment, calculations, attention span, abstract thinking; agnosia	Difficulty concentrating, forgetfulness, inattention
Level of consciousness	Altered	Not altered	Not altered

Continued

TABLE 2.2	Delirium, Dementia, and Depression—cont'd		
	Delirium	**Dementia**	**Depression**
Activity level	Can be increased or reduced; restlessness; behaviors may worsen in evening (sundowning); sleep/wake cycle may be reversed	Not altered; behaviors may worsen in evening (sundowning)	Usually decreased; lethargy, fatigue, lack of motivation; may sleep poorly and awaken in early morning
Emotional state	Rapid swings; can be fearful, anxious, suspicious, aggressive, have hallucinations and/ or delusions	Flat; agitation	Extreme sadness, apathy, irritability, anxiety, paranoid ideation
Speech and language	Rapid, inappropriate, incoherent, rambling	Incoherent, slow (sometimes due to effort to find the right word), inappropriate, rambling, repetitious	Slow, flat, low
Prognosis	Reversible with proper and timely treatment	Not reversible; progressive	Reversible with proper and timely treatment

From Halter, M. J. (2014). *Varcarolis' foundations of psychiatric mental health nursing* (7th ed.). St. Louis: Elsevier.

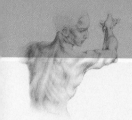

CHAPTER 3

Assessment Techniques and Safety in the Clinical Setting

ASSESSMENT TECHNIQUES

The skills requisite for the physical examination are inspection, palpation, percussion, and auscultation. The skills are performed one at a time and in this order.

Inspection

Inspection is close, careful scrutiny, first of the person as a whole and then of each body system. Inspection begins the moment you first meet the individual and develop a "general survey." (Specific data to consider for the general survey are presented in the following chapter.) As you proceed through the examination, start the assessment of each body system with inspection.

Learn to use each person as his or her own control and compare the right and left sides of the body. The two sides are nearly symmetric. Inspection requires good lighting, adequate exposure, and occasional use of instruments (otoscope, ophthalmoscope, penlight, nasal and vaginal specula) to enlarge or enhance your view.

Palpation

Palpation follows and often confirms points that you noted during inspection. Palpation applies your sense of touch to assess these factors: texture; temperature; moisture; organ location and size; and any swelling, vibration or pulsation, rigidity or spasticity, crepitation, presence of lumps or masses, and presence of tenderness or pain. Different parts of the hands are best suited for assessing different factors:

- Fingertips—Best for fine tactile discrimination such as skin texture, swelling, pulsatility, and presence of lumps
- A grasping action of the fingers and thumb—To detect the position, shape, and consistency of an organ or mass
- The dorsa (backs) of hands and fingers—Best for determining temperature because the skin here is thinner than on the palms
- Base of fingers (metacarpophalangeal joints) or ulnar surface of the hand—To detect vibration

Your palpation technique should be slow and systematic. Warm your hands by kneading them together or holding them under warm water. Identify any tender areas and palpate them last.

Start with light palpation to detect surface characteristics and accustom the person to being touched.

When deep palpation is needed (as for abdominal contents), intermittent pressure is better than one long, continuous palpation. Avoid any situation in which continuous or deep palpation could cause internal injury or pain.

Bimanual palpation requires the use of both hands to envelop or capture certain body parts or organs such as the kidneys, uterus, or adnexa for more precise delimitation.

Percussion

Percussion involves tapping the person's skin with short, sharp strokes to assess underlying structures. The strokes yield a palpable vibration and a characteristic sound that depicts the location, size, and density of the underlying organ.

The Stationary Hand. Hyperextend the middle finger of your nondominant hand (the pleximeter) and place its distal portion *firmly* against the person's skin. Avoid the ribs and scapulae. Percussing over a bone yields no data because it always sounds "dull." Lift the rest of the stationary hand up off the person's skin (Fig. 3.1); otherwise the resting hand will dampen off the produced vibrations just as a drummer uses the hand to halt a drum roll.

The Striking Hand. Use the middle finger of your dominant hand as the *striking* finger (the plexor). Hold your forearm close to the skin surface

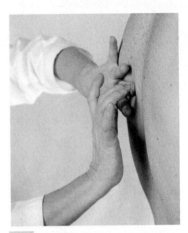

3.1 Percussion.

with your upper arm and shoulder steady but not rigid. The action is all in the wrist, and it *must* be relaxed.

Bounce your middle finger off the stationary one. Aim for just behind the nail bed. Flex the striking finger so that its tip, not the finger pad, makes

TABLE 3.1	Characteristics of Percussion Notes		
Type	Amplitude	Pitch	Quality
Resonant	Medium loud	Low	Clear, hollow
Hyperresonant	Louder	Lower	Booming
Tympany	Loud	High	Musical and drumlike (like a kettle drum)
Dull	Soft	High	Muffled thud
Flat	Very soft	High	A dead stop of sound; absolute dullness

contact. It hits directly at right angles to the stationary finger.

Percuss two times in each location using even, staccato blows. Lift the striking finger off quickly; a resting finger dampens vibrations. Then move to a new body location and repeat, keeping your technique even (Table 3.1).

Auscultation

Auscultation is listening to sounds produced by the body such as the heart, blood vessels, lungs, and abdomen through a **stethoscope**.

Choose a stethoscope with two endpieces—a diaphragm and a bell. The **diaphragm** has a flat edge and is best for high-pitched sounds—breath, bowel, and normal heart sounds. Hold the diaphragm firmly against the person's skin, firmly enough to leave a slight ring afterward.

The **bell** endpiece has a deep, hollow, cuplike shape. It is best for soft, low-pitched sounds such as extra heart sounds or murmurs. Hold it lightly against the person's skin, just enough so it forms a perfect seal. Pressing harder causes the skin to act as a diaphragm, obliterating the low-pitched sounds.

Some newer stethoscopes have one endpiece with a "tunable diaphragm." This enables you to listen to both low- and high-frequency sounds without rotation of the endpiece.

SETTING

- The examination room should be warm and comfortable, quiet, private, and well lit.
- When possible, stop any distracting noises.
- Discourage interruptions.
- Lighting with natural daylight is best, although artificial light will suffice.
- Position a wall or standing lamp for high-intensity lighting.

Duration	Sample Location
Moderate	Over normal lung tissue
Longer	Normal over a child's lung; in an adult over lungs with abnormal amount of air such as in emphysema
Sustained longest	Over air-filled viscus (e.g., the stomach, the intestine)
Short	Over relatively dense organs (e.g., liver and spleen)
Very short	When no air is present or over thigh muscles, bone, or tumor

- The examination table is positioned so both sides are easily accessible and at a height at which you can stand without stooping.
- The table should be equipped to raise the patient's head up to 45 degrees.
- A roll-up stool is needed for the sections of the examination for which you must be sitting.
- A bedside table should be nearby to allow you to lay out your equipment.

EQUIPMENT

Before the examination have all your equipment within easy reach and laid out in an organized manner. These items are usually needed for a complete physical examination:

Platform scale with height attachment
Sphygmomanometer
Stethoscope with bell and diaphragm endpieces
Thermometer
Pulse oximeter (in hospital setting)
Paper and pencil or pen
Flashlight or penlight
Otoscope/ophthalmoscope
Tuning fork
Tongue depressor
Pocket vision screener
Skin marking pen
Flexible tape measure and ruler marked in centimeters
Reflex hammer
Sharp object (sterile needle or split-tongue blade)
Cotton balls
Bivalve vaginal speculum
Clean gloves
Materials for cytologic study
Lubricant
Fecal occult blood test materials

A SAFER ENVIRONMENT

Designate a "clean" versus a "used" area for handling of your equipment. Distinguish the clean area by one or two disposable paper towels. On the towels place all the single-use, newly cleaned, or newly alcohol-wiped equipment that you will use on this patient.

Equipment that is used frequently on many patients can become a common vehicle for transmission of infection. Use alcohol wipes to clean all equipment that you carry from patient to patient, e.g., your stethoscope endpieces, the reflex hammer, or ruler. As you proceed through the examination, pick up each piece of equipment from the clean area and, after use on the patient, relegate it to the used area or throw it directly into the trash.

Take all steps to avoid any possible transmission of infection between patients or between patient and examiner. The single most important step to decrease risk of microorganism transmission is to wash your hands promptly and thoroughly (Table 3.2). Using alcohol-based hand rubs takes less time than soap-and-water handwashing; it also kills more organisms more quickly and is less damaging to the skin because of emollients added to the product. Use the mechanical action of soap-and-water handwashing when hands are visibly soiled and when patients are infected with spore-forming organisms (e.g., *Clostridium difficile*).

APPROACH TO THE CLINICAL SETTING

Preparation for a Complete Assessment

Most people, whether entering the hospital or receiving outpatient care, initially require a complete physical examination. Before you begin, ask the person to empty his or her bladder and save a urine specimen if needed.

Begin by measuring the person's height, weight, blood pressure, temperature, pulse, and respirations. If

TABLE 3.2	Standard and Universal Precautions for Use With All Patients

STANDARD PRECAUTIONS are based on the principle that all blood, body fluids, secretions, excretions (except sweat), nonintact skin, and mucous membranes may contain transmissible infectious agents. Precautions apply to all patients, regardless of suspected or confirmed infection status, and in any setting in which health care is delivered. Components are:

Hand hygiene. (1) Avoid unnecessary touching of surfaces in close proximity to the patient; (2) when hands are visibly dirty, contaminated with proteinaceous material, or visibly soiled with blood or body fluids, wash hands with soap and water; (3) if not visibly soiled, decontaminate hands with an alcohol-based hand rub. Perform hand hygiene: (a) before having direct contact with patients; (b) after contact with blood, body fluids or excretions, mucous membranes, nonintact skin, or wound dressings; (c) after contact with a patient's intact skin (e.g., taking a pulse or blood pressure or lifting a patient); (d) after contact with medical equipment in the immediate vicinity of the patient; (e) after removing gloves.

Use of gloves, gown, mask, eye protection, or face shield. (1) Wear gloves when you anticipate that contact with blood or other potentially infectious materials, mucous membranes, nonintact skin, or potentially contaminated intact skin (e.g., patient incontinent of stool or urine) could occur. (2) Wear a gown to protect skin and clothing when you anticipate contact with blood, body fluids, secretions, or excretions. (3) Use mouth, nose, and eye protection to protect the mucous membranes during procedures that are likely to generate splashes or sprays of blood, body fluids, secretions, and excretions.

Respiratory hygiene/cough etiquette is targeted at patients and accompanying people with undiagnosed transmissible respiratory infections. Elements include: (1) education of staff, patients, and visitors; (2) posted signs in language(s) appropriate to the population; (3) source control measures (e.g., covering the mouth/nose with a tissue when coughing and promptly disposing of used tissues, using surgical masks on the coughing person); (4) hand hygiene after contact with respiratory secretions; and (5) spatial separation of more than 3 feet of people with respiratory infections in common waiting areas.

Modified from Centers for Disease Control and Prevention. (2007). *Preventing transmissions of infectious agents in healthcare settings*. http://www.cdc.gov/hicpac/2007IP/2007isolationPrecautions.html.

needed, measure visual acuity at this time using the Snellen eye chart.

Ask the person to change into an examining gown, leaving the underwear on. Unless your assistance is needed, leave the room as the person undresses.

Consider safety and protect yourself and the patient against the spread of any possible infection. As you reenter the room, wash your hands in the person's presence. This indicates that you are protective of the patient and are starting fresh for him or her. Wear gloves when there is potential contact with any body fluids (e.g., mouth or genitalia examination).

Explain each step in the examination and how the person can cooperate. Encourage him or her to ask questions. Keep your own movements slow, methodic, and deliberate.

As you proceed through the examination, avoid distractions and concentrate on one step at a time. The sequence of the steps may differ, depending on the age of the patient and your own preference; however, you should establish a system that works for you and stick to it to avoid omissions.

Organize the steps so the person does not change positions too often. Although proper exposure is necessary, use additional drapes to maintain the person's privacy and prevent chilling.

(See Chapter 20 for the sequence of steps in the complete physical examination.)

The Sick Person

For the ill person in some distress, alter the position during the examination. For example, a patient with shortness of breath or ear pain may want to sit up, whereas a person with faintness or overwhelming fatigue may want to be supine. Initially it may be necessary just to examine the body areas appropriate to the problem, collecting a *focused* or *mini database*. You may return to finish a complete assessment after the initial distress is resolved.

Focused or Problem-Centered Assessment

This is for a limited or short-term problem. Here you collect a focused database, smaller in scope than the complete assessment. It concerns mainly one problem, one cue complex, or one body system. It is used in all settings—hospital, primary care, and long-term care.

Follow-up Assessment

The status of any identified problems should be evaluated at regular and appropriate intervals. What change has occurred? Is the problem getting better or worse? Which coping strategies are used? This type of assessment is used in all settings to follow up short-term or chronic health problems.

For more information on the preparation of infants, children, and older adults for the physical examination, see Jarvis: *Physical Examination and Health Assessment,* 8th ed.

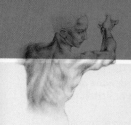

CHAPTER 4

General Survey, Measurement, Vital Signs, and Pain Assessment

GENERAL SURVEY

The general survey is a study of the whole person, covering the general health state and any obvious physical characteristics. Begin building a general survey from the moment you first encounter the person. What leaves an immediate impression?

As you proceed through the health history, the measurements, and the vital signs, note the following points, which will add up to the general survey: physical appearance, body structure, mobility, and behavior.

PHYSICAL APPEARANCE

Age—The person appears to be his or her stated age.

Sexual development—Development is appropriate for sex and age.

Level of consciousness—The person is alert and oriented, attends to questions, and responds appropriately.

Skin color—Color tone is even, pigmentation varying with genetic background; skin is intact with no obvious lesions.

Facial features—Features are symmetric with movement.

There are no signs of acute distress.

BODY STRUCTURE

Stature—The height appears within normal range for age and genetic heritage.

Nutrition—The weight appears within normal range for height and body build. Body fat distribution is even.

Symmetry—Body parts look equal bilaterally and are in relative proportion to one another.

Posture—The person stands comfortably erect as appropriate for age.

Position—The person sits comfortably in a chair or on the bed or examination table, with arms relaxed at sides and head turned to examiner.

Body build, contour—Proportions are:
1. Arm span (fingertip to fingertip) equals height.
2. Body length from crown to pubis is roughly equal to length from pubis to sole.

Obvious physical deformities—Note any congenital or acquired defects.

MOBILITY

Gait—Normally the base is as wide as the shoulder width. Foot placement is accurate. The walk is smooth, even, and well balanced; associated movements such as symmetric arm swing are present.

Range of motion—Note full mobility for each joint and whether movement is deliberate, accurate, smooth, and coordinated. No involuntary movement is present.

BEHAVIOR

Facial expression—The person maintains eye contact (unless there is a cultural taboo). Expressions are appropriate to the situation.

Mood and affect—The person is cooperative with the examiner and interacts pleasantly.

Speech—Articulation (the ability to form words) is clear and understandable. The stream of speech is fluent, with an even pace. Ideas are conveyed clearly. Word choice is appropriate to culture and education. The person communicates in prevailing language easily by himself or herself or with an interpreter.

Dress—Clothing is appropriate to the climate, looks clean and fits the body, and is appropriate to the person's culture and age-group.

Personal hygiene—The person appears clean and groomed appropriately for his or her age, occupation, and socioeconomic group. Hair is groomed or brushed. Makeup is appropriate for age and culture.

MEASUREMENT

WEIGHT

Use a standardized *balance* or *electronic scale*. Instruct the person to remove his or her shoes and heavy outer clothing before standing on the scale. When a sequence of repeated weights is necessary, aim for approximately the same time of day and the same type of clothing worn each time. Record the weight in kilograms and pounds.

Compare the person's weight with the previous health visit. A recent weight loss may be explained by dieting. An unexplained weight loss may be a sign of a short-term illness (e.g., fever, infection, disease of the mouth or throat) or a chronic illness (endocrine disease, malignancy, mental health dysfunction).

A weight gain usually reflects overabundant caloric intake, unhealthy eating habits, or a sedentary lifestyle.

Obesity, or the excessive accumulation of fat in the body, is more than 120% of ideal weight with regard to age, height, and body structure. Occasionally obesity may be caused by endocrine disorders, drug therapy (e.g., corticosteroids), or depression.

HEIGHT

Use a wall-mounted device or the measuring pole on the balance scale. Align the extended headpiece with the top of the head. The person should be shoeless, standing straight, and looking straight ahead. Heels, buttocks, and shoulders should be in contact with a hard surface.

Arm Span or Total Arm Length

Measurement of arm span is useful for situations in which height is difficult to measure such as in children with cerebral palsy or scoliosis or in older adults with spinal curvature. Arm span, which is nearly equivalent to height, is sometimes used clinically instead of height.

Ask the person to hold the arms straight out from the sides of the body. Measure the distance from the tip of the middle finger on one hand to the tip of the middle finger on the other hand.

BODY MASS INDEX

Body mass index (BMI) is a practical marker of optimal healthy weight for height and an indicator of obesity or malnutrition. BMI expresses the relationship between height and weight but does not consider other variables, such as muscle mass. BMI also may be less useful in children or in older adults. Researchers recommend using BMI in conjunction with other measures, such as waist circumference (Nazare et al., 2015).

A healthy BMI is a level of 19 to less than 25. Show the person how his or her own weight matches up to the national guidelines for optimal BMI. Note that BMI overestimates body fat in people who are very muscular, and it underestimates body fat in older adults who have lost muscle mass.

BMI classifications for adults are as follows:

Underweight: less than 18.5 kg/m^2
Normal weight: 18.5 to 24.9 kg/m^2
Overweight: 25 to 29.9 kg/m^2
Obesity (Class 1): 30 to 34.9 kg/m^2
Obesity (Class 2): 35 to 39.9 kg/m^2
Extreme obesity (Class 3): ≥40 kg/m^2

WAIST CIRCUMFERENCE

Excess abdominal fat is an important, independent risk factor for disease, over and above that of BMI. With the person standing, locate the hip bone and the top of its iliac crest. Place a measuring tape around the waist parallel to the floor at the level of the iliac crest. The tape should be snug but not pinch in the skin. Note the measurement at the end of a normal expiration (Fig. 4.1). A waist circumference (WC) of 35

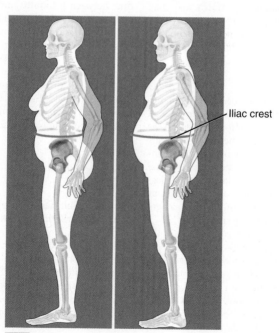

Iliac crest

4.1 Measuring-tape position for abdominal circumference. (© Pat Thomas, 2010.)

inches or more in women and 40 inches or more in men increases the risk for type 2 diabetes, dyslipidemia, hypertension, and cardiovascular disease (CVD) in people with a BMI between 25 and 35 kg/m².

DEVELOPMENTAL COMPETENCE

Infants and Children

Weight

Weigh an infant on a platform-type balance scale. To check calibration, set the weight at zero and observe the beam balance. Guard the baby so he or she does not fall. Weigh to the nearest 10 g (½ oz) for infants and 100 g (¼ lb) for toddlers.

By age 2 or 3 years use the upright scale. Leave underpants on the child. Some young children are fearful of the rickety standing platform and may prefer sitting on the infant scale. Use the upright scale with preschoolers and school-age children, maintaining modesty with light clothing.

Length

Until age 2 years measure the infant's body length supine with a horizontal measuring board. Hold the head in the midline. Because the infant normally has flexed legs, extend them momentarily by holding the knees together and pushing them down until the legs are flat on the table. Avoid using a tape measure along the infant's length because this is inaccurate.

By age 2 or 3 years measure the child's height by standing him or her against the pole on the platform scale or against a flat ruler taped to the wall. Encourage the child to stand straight and tall and look straight ahead without tilting the head. The shoulders, buttocks, and heels should touch the wall. Hold a book or flat board on the child's head at a right angle to the wall. Mark just under the book or board, noting the measure to the nearest 1 mm (⅛ inch).

Head Circumference

Measure the infant's head circumference at birth and at each well-child visit up to age 2 years and then annually up to age 6 years. Circle the tape around the head at the prominent frontal and occipital bones; the widest span is correct. Plot the measurement on standardized growth charts. Compare the infant's head size with that expected for age. A series of measurements is more valuable than a single figure to show the *rate* of head growth.

A newborn's head measures about 32 to 38 cm (average about 34 cm) and is about 2 cm larger than the chest circumference. The chest grows at a faster rate than the cranium; at some time between 6 months and 2 years both measurements are about the same; after age 2 the chest circumference is greater than the head circumference.

Measurement of the chest circumference is valuable as a comparison with the head circumference but is not necessarily valuable by itself. Circle the tape around the chest at the nipple line. It should be snug but not so tight as to leave a mark.

The Aging Adult

Weight

An older adult has more prominent bony landmarks than a younger adult. Body weight decreases during the 70s and 80s. This factor is more evident in males, perhaps because of greater muscle shrinkage. The distribution of fat also changes when people are in their 70s and 80s. Subcutaneous fat is lost from the face and periphery (especially the forearms), and additional fat is deposited in the abdomen and hips.

Height

By their 70s and 80s many people are shorter than they were in their 60s. This results from thinning of the vertebral discs and shortening of the individual vertebrae as postural changes of kyphosis and slight flexion in the knees and hips. Because long bones do not shorten with age, the overall body proportion appears different—a shorter trunk with relatively long extremities.

Kyphosis is an exaggerated posterior curvature of the thoracic spine (hump-back). See Table 19.3, p. 434, in Jarvis: *Physical Examination and Health Assessment,* 8th ed.

VITAL SIGNS

TEMPERATURE

The normal oral temperature in a resting person is 37°C (98.6°F), with a range of 35.8° to 37.3°C (96.4° to 99.1°F). The rectal temperature measures 0.5°C (1°F) higher. The normal temperature is influenced by:

- A diurnal cycle of 1° to 1.5°F, with the trough occurring in the early morning hours and the peak occurring in late afternoon to early evening.
- The menstruation cycle in women. Progesterone secretion, occurring with ovulation at midcycle, causes a 0.5° to 1.0°F rise in temperature that continues until menses.
- Exercise. Moderate-to-hard exercise increases body temperature.
- Age. Wider normal variations occur in infants and young children because of less effective heat-control mechanisms. In older adults temperature is usually lower than in other age-groups, with a mean of 36.2°C (97.2°F).

The **tympanic membrane thermometer** (TMT) and **temporal artery thermometer** (TAT) are noninvasive, nontraumatic devices that provide rapid temperature readings. The TMT probe tip is shaped like an otoscope. Gently place the covered probe tip in the ear canal. Do not force it and do not occlude the canal. Activate the device and read the temperature in 2 seconds (Fig. 4.2). The TAT uses infrared emissions to obtain the temperature reading. To use the TAT, slide the device across the forehead ending behind the ear. The reading should take 6 seconds or less.

The **electronic thermometer** has the advantages of swift and accurate measurements (usually within 30 seconds) and of being safe and unbreakable. The instrument must be fully charged and correctly calibrated. Read the instructions carefully before use. Electronic thermometers can be used for both oral and rectal temperatures. Blue-tipped probes are for the oral route, whereas red-tipped probes are rectal.

Shake the **glass thermometer** down to 35.5°C (96°F) and place it at the

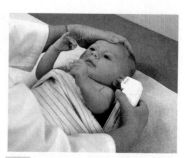

4.2

base of the tongue in either of the posterior sublingual pockets, *not* in front of the tongue. Instruct the person to keep his or her lips closed. Leave in place 3 to 4 minutes if the person is afebrile and up to 8 minutes if febrile. Wait 15 minutes before inserting the thermometer if the person has just taken hot or iced liquids and 2 minutes if he or she has just smoked.

Take a **rectal** temperature only when the other routes are not practical, such as for people who are comatose or confused, in shock, or unable to close the mouth. Wear gloves and insert a lubricated rectal thermometer 2 to 3 cm (1 inch) into the adult rectum, directed toward the umbilicus. Do not let go of the temperature probe while it is inserted into the rectum. (Note that a glass thermometer registers in $2\frac{1}{2}$ minutes.)

PULSE

Using the pads of your first three fingers, palpate the radial pulse at the flexor aspect of the wrist laterally along the radius bone. Push until you feel the strongest pulsation. If the rhythm is regular, count the number of beats in 30 seconds and multiply by 2. However, if the rhythm is irregular, count for 1 full minute. As you begin the counting interval, start your count with "zero" for the first pulse felt. The second pulse felt is "one," and so on (Hollerbach & Sneed, 1990).

In a resting adult the normal heart rate range is 50 to 95 bpm (beats/min), and well-conditioned athletes may have a resting rate less than 50 bpm. The rate normally varies with age, being more rapid in infancy and childhood (Table 4.1) and more moderate during adulthood and older years. The rate also varies with sex; after puberty females have a slightly faster rate than males.

RESPIRATIONS

Normally a person's breathing is relaxed, regular, automatic, and silent. Most people are unaware of their breathing; therefore do not mention that you will be counting the respirations because sudden awareness may alter the normal pattern. Instead maintain your position of counting the radial pulse and unobtrusively count the respirations. Count for 30 seconds if respirations are normal or for 1 full minute if you suspect an abnormality. Avoid the 15-second interval because the result can vary by a factor of ±4, which is significant with such a small number.

Respiratory rates are 10 to 20 breaths/min for adults and are normally more rapid for infants and

TABLE 4.1	Normal Heart Rate (Beats Per Minute) in Infants and Children		
Age	Resting (Awake)	Resting (Asleep)	Exercise/Fever
Newborn	100-180	80-160	Up to 220
1 wk-3 mo	100-220	80-200	Up to 220
3 mo-2 yr	80-150	70-120	Up to 220
2-10 yr	70-100	60-90	195-215
10-20 yr	55-90	50-90	195-215

Adapted from Burns, C. E., Dunn, A. M., Brady, M. A., et al. (2013). *Pediatric primary care* (5th ed.). Philadelphia: Elsevier.

TABLE 4.2	Normal Respiratory Rates
Age (Yr)	Respiratory Rate (Breaths/Minute)
0-1	24-38
1-3	22-30
4-6	20-24
7-9	18-24
10-14	16-22
15-18	14-20
Adult	10-20

Adapted from Burns, C. E., Dunn, A. M., Brady, M. A., et al. (2013). *Pediatric primary care* (5th ed.). Philadelphia: Elsevier.

children (Table 4.2). A fairly constant ratio of pulse rate to respiratory rate is about 4:1. Normally both pulse and respiratory rates rise in response to exercise or anxiety.

BLOOD PRESSURE

Blood pressure (BP) is the force of the blood pushing against the side of the vessel wall. The **systolic** pressure is the maximum pressure felt on the artery during left ventricular contraction, or systole. The **diastolic** pressure is the resting pressure that the blood constantly exerts between each contraction. The **pulse pressure** is the difference between the systolic and diastolic pressures and reflects the stroke volume.

BP varies normally with many factors:

Age: Normally there is a gradual rise through childhood and into adult years.

Sex: Before puberty there is no difference between males and females. After puberty females usually show a lower BP reading than their male counterparts. After menopause BP in females is higher than in their male counterparts.

Race: In the United States a black adult's BP is usually higher than that of a white adult of the same age. The incidence of hypertension is twice as high in blacks as in whites. The reasons for this appear to be genetic heritage and environmental factors.

Diurnal rhythm: There is a daily cycle of a peak and a trough. BP climbs to a high in late afternoon or early evening and then declines to an early-morning low.

Weight: BP is higher in obese people than in people of normal weight of the same age (including adolescents).

Exercise: Increasing activity yields a proportionate increase in BP. Within 5 minutes of terminating exercise, BP normally returns to baseline.

Emotions: BP momentarily rises with fear, anger, and pain as a result of stimulation of the sympathetic nervous system.

Stress: BP is elevated in people experiencing continual tension because of lifestyle, occupational stress, or life problems.

Blood pressure is measured with a stethoscope and a *sphygmomanometer*. The cuff consists of an inflatable rubber bladder inside a cloth cover. The width of the rubber bladder should equal 40% of the circumference of the extremity used. The length of the bladder should equal 80% of the arm circumference.

The size is important; using a cuff that is too narrow yields a falsely high BP. Match the appropriate-size cuff to the person's arm size and shape and not to his or her age.

Arm Pressure. A comfortable, relaxed person yields a valid BP. Many people are anxious at the beginning of an examination; allow at least a 5-minute rest before measuring the BP.

The patient may be sitting or lying with the bare arm supported at the heart level. Palpate the brachial artery, which is located just above the antecubital fossa medially. With the cuff deflated, center it about 2.5 cm (1 inch) above the brachial artery and wrap it evenly.

Now palpate the brachial or radial artery. Inflate the cuff until the artery pulsation is obliterated. Note that number. Deflate the cuff quickly and completely; then wait 15 to 30 seconds before reinflating so the blood trapped in the veins can dissipate. When you inflate the cuff to auscultate the blood pressure, you will add 20 to 30 mm Hg to identify the maximal inflation level. This avoids missing an **auscultatory gap**, which is a period when Korotkoff sounds disappear during auscultation and is common in hypertension.

Place the stethoscope over the site of the brachial artery, making a light but airtight seal (Fig. 4.3). Inflate the cuff to the maximal inflation level; then deflate the cuff slowly and evenly (2 mm Hg/heartbeat). Note the points at which you hear the first appearance of sound (the systolic pressure value), the muffling of sound, and the

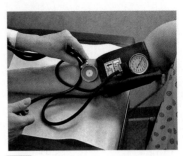

4.3

final disappearance of sound. These are phases I, IV, and V of *Korotkoff sounds.*

In children and adults phase V (the last audible sound) indicates diastolic pressure. However, when a variance greater than 10 to 12 mm Hg exists between phases IV and V, record *both* phases along with the systolic reading (e.g., 142/98/80). Clear communication is important because results significantly affect diagnosis and planning of care. Table 4.3 presents a list of common errors in BP measurement.

TABLE 4.3	Common Sources of Error in Blood Pressure Measurement

Errors that produce a falsely *high* reading:
- Failure to use the appropriate cuff size; a too-narrow cuff gives a higher reading
- Wrapping the cuff too loosely or unevenly; cuff pressure must be exceedingly high to compress the brachial artery
- Recording blood pressure just after a meal, while person is smoking, or while person's bladder is distended
- Deflating the cuff too slowly; this produces venous congestion in the extremity, which falsely elevates diastolic pressure

Errors that produce a falsely *low* reading:
- Having the person's arm above the level of the heart (effect of hydrostatic pressure can give an error up to 10 mm Hg in systolic and diastolic pressure)
- Failure to notice an auscultatory gap
- Diminished hearing acuity of the health care professional
- Stethoscope that is too small or too large or has tubing that is too long
- Inability to hear feeble Korotkoff sounds

Errors that produce *either* falsely *high* or *low* readings:
- Inaccurately calibrated manometer
- Defective equipment (e.g., valve, connections)
- Performing the technique too quickly, with too little attention to details

If the person is known to have hypertension, is taking antihypertensive medications, or reports a history of fainting or syncope, take the BP reading with him or her in three positions—lying down, sitting, and standing. Normally a slight decrease (less than 10 mm Hg) in systolic pressure may occur when the position is changed from supine to standing.

Orthostatic hypotension, a drop in systolic pressure of more than 20 mm Hg, may occur with a quick change to a standing position. It is caused by abrupt peripheral vasodilation without a compensatory increase in cardiac output. Older people have the greatest risk of this problem. It also occurs with prolonged bed rest, hypovolemia, and some medications. Table 4.4 presents further information on hypotension and hypertension.

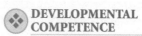 **DEVELOPMENTAL COMPETENCE**

The aorta and major arteries tend to harden with age. As the heart pumps against a stiffer aorta, the systolic pressure increases, leading to a widened pulse pressure. With many older people both the systolic and diastolic pressures increase, making it difficult to distinguish normal aging values from abnormal hypertension.

THE DOPPLER TECHNIQUE

The Doppler technique is used to locate peripheral pulse sites. For BP measurement, the Doppler technique augments Korotkoff sounds when they are hard to hear with a stethoscope such as in critically ill people with a low BP, infants with small arms, and obese

TABLE 4.4	Abnormalities in Blood Pressure

HYPOTENSION

In normotensive adults	Below 95/60 mm Hg
In hypertensive adults	Below the person's average reading but above 95/60 mm Hg
In children	Below expected value for age

Occurs With	Rationale
Acute myocardial infarction	Decreased cardiac output
Shock	Decreased cardiac output
Hemorrhage	Decrease in total blood volume
Vasodilation	Decrease in peripheral vascular resistance
Addison's disease (hypofunction of adrenal glands)	

Associated Symptoms and Signs

In conditions of decreased cardiac output, a low blood pressure is accompanied by an increased pulse, dizziness, diaphoresis, confusion, and blurred vision. The skin feels cool and clammy because the superficial blood vessels constrict to shunt blood to the vital organs. An individual having an acute myocardial infarction may also complain of crushing substernal chest pain, high epigastric pain, and shoulder or jaw pain.

HYPERTENSION
Essential or Primary Hypertension
This occurs from no known cause but is responsible for about 95% of cases of hypertension in adults.

Continued

Summary of Blood Pressure Guidelines

	Target BP	Initial Treatment	Special Considerations
ACC/AHA Task Force[a]	<130/80 mm Hg	In patients without cardiovascular disease (CVD) and 10-year atherosclerotic CVD risk of <10%, begin treatment ≥140/90 mm Hg In patients with CVD or 10-year atherosclerotic CVD risk ≥10%, begin treatment ≥130/80 mm Hg	Consider lower BP targets for high-risk individuals such as those with diabetes or chronic kidney disease (CKD).
JNC-8 Guidelines[b]	Adults ≥60 yr, less than 150/90 mm Hg Adults <60 yr with diabetes or CKD, less than 140/90 mm Hg	Lifestyle modification and pharmacologic therapy beginning with thiazide diuretics, CCB, ACEI, or ARB in non–African-American patients	Initial treatment for African-American patients is a CCB or a thiazide diuretic. CKD patients should begin with an ACEI or ARB.

ACEI, Angiotensin-converting enzyme inhibitor; *ARB,* angiotensin II receptor blocker; *CCB,* calcium channel blocker.
[a]Whelton, P. K., Carey, R. M., Aronow, W. S., et al. (2017). 2017 ACC/AHA/AAPA/ABC/ACPM/AGS/APhA/ ASH/ASPC/NMA/PCNA Guideline for the prevention, detection, evaluation, and management of high blood pressure in adults. *J Am Coll Cardiol.* doi:10.1016/j.jacc.2017.11.006.
[b]James, P. A., Oparil, S., & Carter, B. L. (2014). 2014 Evidence-based guidelines for the management of high blood pressure in adults: report from the panel members appointed to the Eighth Joint National Committee (JNC 8). *JAMA, 311,* 507-520.

people in whom the sounds are muffled by layers of fat. Proper cuff placement is also difficult on an obese person's cone-shaped upper arm. In this situation you can place the cuff on the more even forearm and hold the Doppler probe over the radial artery (Fig. 4.4). For either location use this procedure:

- Apply coupling gel to the transducer probe.
- Turn the Doppler probe on.
- Touch the probe to the skin, holding the probe perpendicular to the artery.
- A pulsatile whooshing sound indicates location of the artery. You may need to rotate the probe, but maintain contact with the skin. Do not push the probe too hard or you will wipe out the pulse.
- Inflate the cuff until the sounds disappear; then proceed another 20 to 30 mm Hg beyond that point.
- Slowly deflate the cuff, noting the point at which the first whooshing

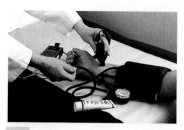

4.4 Measuring blood pressure using the Doppler technique.

sounds appear. This is the systolic pressure.

- It is difficult to hear the muffling of sound or a reliable disappearance of sounds indicating the diastolic pressure (phases IV and V of Korotkoff sounds). However, the systolic blood pressure alone gives valuable data on the level of tissue perfusion and blood flow through patent vessels.

PAIN ASSESSMENT

Pain is a highly complex and subjective experience that originates from the central (CNS), the peripheral nervous system (PNS), or both. Pain is defined as "an unpleasant sensory and emotional experience associated with actual or potential tissue damage, or described in terms of such damage" (International Association for the Study of Pain, 2018). Pain is a subjective experience, and as such the person's report is the most reliable indicator of pain. With knowledge that pain occurs on a neurochemical level, the clinician cannot base the diagnosis of pain exclusively on physical exam findings. Physical exam findings can lend support. At this time x-ray images, computed tomography (CT) scans, and magnetic resonance images (MRIs) are not sensitive enough to identify minute damage to nerve fibers.

Pain is multidimensional in scope, encompassing physical, affective, and functional domains. Various tools have been developed to capture unidimensional aspects (e.g., intensity) or multidimensional components. Select the pain assessment tool based on its purpose, time involved in administration, and the patient's ability to comprehend and complete the tool.

Pain Rating Scales are unidimensional and are intended to reflect pain intensity. They come in various forms. They can indicate a baseline intensity, track changes, and give some degree of evaluation to a treatment modality. **Numeric Rating Scales** ask the patient to choose a number that rates the level of pain, with 0 indicating no pain and 10 indicating the worst pain. It can be administered verbally or visually along a vertical or horizontal line (Fig. 4.5).

 DEVELOPMENTAL COMPETENCE

Infants

Infants have the same capacity for pain as adults. Preverbal infants are at high risk for undertreatment of pain because of persistent myths and beliefs that infants do not remember pain. Infants are incapable of self-report, so pain assessment relies on behavioral and

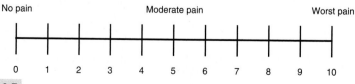

No pain   Moderate pain   Worst pain

0   1   2   3   4   5   6   7   8   9   10

4.5

physiologic clues. The FLACC (Face, Legs, Activity, Cry, Consolability) scale can be used to measure pain in infants and young children.

Children 2 years of age can report pain and point to its location. They cannot rate pain intensity at this developmental level. It is helpful to ask the parent or caregiver which words his or her child uses to report pain (e.g., boo-boo, owie). Some children will try to be "grown-up and brave" and often deny having pain in the presence of a stranger or if they are fearful of receiving a "shot."

Rating scales can be introduced at 4 or 5 years of age. The Faces Pain Scale–Revised is one example; the child is asked to choose a face that shows "how much you hurt (right now)." (See Jarvis: *Physical Examination and Health Assessment,* 8th ed., p. 169.)

The Aging Adult

No evidence exists to suggest that older individuals perceive pain to a lesser degree or that sensitivity is diminished. Although pain is a common experience among individuals 65 years of age and older, it is *not* a normal process of aging. Pain indicates pathology/injury. It should never be considered something to tolerate or accept in one's later years.

People with dementia become less able to identify and describe pain over time, although pain is still present and destructive. They communicate pain through their behavior. Agitation, pacing, and repetitive yelling may indicate pain and not a worsening of the dementia.

In general, older adults find the numeric scale to be abstract and have difficulty responding, especially with a fluctuating chronic pain experience. An alternative is the simple **Descriptor Scale** that lists words that describe different levels of pain intensity such as *no pain, mild pain, moderate pain,* and *severe pain.* Older adults often respond to scales in which words are selected.

DOCUMENTATION

Sample Charting

K.A. is a 56-year-old male construction worker who appears healthy and of stated age. Alert, oriented, cooperative, with no signs of distress. Ht 170 cm (5′7″). Wt 83 kg (182 lb). BMI 28.5 (overweight). Temp 98.6° F (37°C). Pulse 84 bpm. Resp 14/min. BP 146/84 mm Hg right arm, sitting.

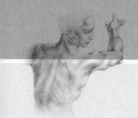

CHAPTER 5

Skin, Hair, and Nails

ANATOMY

Hair shaft

Horny cell layer

Basal cell layer

Melanocyte

Sebaceous gland

Eccrine sweat gland

Apocrine sweat gland

Blood vessels

Adipose tissue

Nerves

Hair follicle

] **Epidermis**

Dermis

Subcutaneous tissue

Connective tissue

Arrector pili muscle

5.1

The skin has two layers—the outer, highly differentiated **epidermis** and the inner supportive **dermis** (Fig. 5.1). The epidermis is stratified into the inner **basal cell layer** that forms new skin cells. It consists of the tough fibrous protein *keratin*. The melanocytes along this layer produce the pigment melanin, which gives brown tones to the skin and hair. From the basal layer the new cells migrate up and flatten into the outer **horny cell layer.** The cells are constantly being shed and replaced with new cells from below.

The **dermis** is the inner supportive layer made up of connective tissue, or *collagen.* This is the tough, fibrous protein that helps the skin resist tearing. It also has elastic tissue that allows the skin to stretch with body movements. Beneath these layers is a third layer—the insulating **subcutaneous** layer of adipose tissue.

The **sebaceous** glands produce a protective lipid, sebum, which is secreted through the hair follicles. The **eccrine** glands are coiled tubules that open directly onto the skin surface and produce the sweat that helps reduce body temperature. The **apocrine** glands open into hair follicles, become active during puberty, and produce sweat with emotional and sexual stimulation.

The **nails** are hard plates of keratin on the dorsal edges of the fingers and

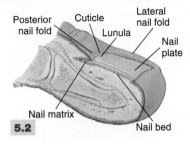

5.2

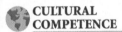

toes (Fig. 5.2). The nail plate is clear, with fine, longitudinal ridges that become prominent with older age. Nails take their pink color from the underlying nail bed of highly vascular epithelial cells.

CULTURAL COMPETENCE

Melanin is responsible for the various colors and tones of skin among people from culturally diverse backgrounds. Melanin protects the skin against harmful ultraviolet rays. The incidence of melanoma is 21 times higher in whites than in Hispanics, and 26 times higher in whites than in blacks. Women outnumber men in melanoma cases before age 50 years, but by age 65 years men have double the rates of women and by age 80 years they are triple (ACS, 2017b). Risk factors are high exposure to ultraviolet (UV) radiation from sunlight or indoor tanning beds, family history of melanoma, and the presence of atypical or numerous (≥50) moles. Risk is increased for persons who sunburn easily or who have natural blond or red hair. Advancing age is a risk because of accumulation of DNA damage over time (Wellbrook, 2016). About 95% of skin melanoma cases are attributable to UV radiation exposure (Islami et al., 2018).

SUBJECTIVE DATA

1. Past history of skin disease (allergies, hives, psoriasis, eczema)
2. Change in pigmentation
3. Change in mole (size or color)
4. Excessive dryness or moisture
5. Pruritus
6. Excessive bruising
7. Rash or lesion
8. Medications (any that cause allergic skin response, increased sunlight sensitivity)
9. Hair loss
10. Change in nails
11. Environmental or occupational hazards (sun exposure, indoor tanning, toxic chemicals, insect bites)
12. Patient-centered care (daily hygiene; use of soaps, cosmetics, or chemicals)

OBJECTIVE DATA

EQUIPMENT NEEDED

Strong direct lighting (natural daylight is ideal to evaluate skin characteristics or use halogen light)
Small centimeter ruler
Lighted magnifier
Gloves

Normal Range of Findings	Abnormal Findings

Inspect and Palpate the Skin

Color

General Pigmentation. The skin tone is consistent with genetic background and varies from pinkish tan to ruddy dark tan, or from light to dark brown, and may have yellow or olive overtones. Dark-skinned people normally have areas of lighter pigmentation on the palms, nail beds, and lips.

General pigmentation is darker in sun-exposed areas. Common (benign) pigmentations also occur:

- **Freckles** (ephelides)—A small, flat increase of brown melanin pigment
- **Nevus** (mole)—A proliferation of melanocytes, tan-to-brown color, flat or raised
- **Birthmarks**—May be tan to brown in color

Advise anyone with moles or birthmarks to perform periodic skin self-examinations. Watch for danger signs listed here. Ask a family member to check any areas that the person cannot see (e.g., the back).

Widespread Color Change. Note any pallor (white), erythema (red), cyanosis (blue), and jaundice (yellow). In dark-skinned people, the amount of normal pigment may mask color changes. Lips and nail beds may not always be accurate signs. The more reliable sites are those with the least pigmentation such as under the tongue, the buccal mucosa, the palpebral conjunctiva, and the sclera. Table 5.1 on pp. 46-47 presents specific clues to assessment.

Temperature

Use the backs (dorsa) of your hands and palpate bilaterally. The skin should be warm with equal temperature bilaterally. Hands and feet may be slightly cooler in a cool environment.

Danger signs: Abnormal characteristics of pigmented lesions are summarized with the mnemonic **ABCDE:**
Asymmetry of a pigmented lesion.
Border irregularity.
Color variation (areas of black, gray, blue, red, white, pink) or dark black.
Diameter greater than 6 mm.
Elevation or evolution.

In addition, report a change in a mole's size, a new pigmented lesion, or the development of itching, burning, or bleeding in a mole. Any of these signs should raise suspicion of malignant melanoma and warrant referral.

Normal Range of Findings	Abnormal Findings
Hypothermia. Generalized coolness may be induced such as in hypothermia used for surgery or high fever. Localized coolness is expected with an immobilized extremity, as when a limb is in a cast or with an intravenous infusion.	General hypothermia accompanies central circulatory disturbance such as with shock. Localized hypothermia occurs in peripheral arterial insufficiency and in Raynaud disease because of vasospasm.
Hyperthermia. Generalized hyperthermia occurs with an increased metabolic rate such as in fever or after heavy exercise. A localized area feels hyperthermic with trauma, infection, or sunburn.	Warm, moist skin occurs with hyperthyroidism as a result of hypermetabolic state.

Moisture

Perspiration appears normally on the face, hands, axilla, and skinfolds in response to activity, a warm environment, or anxiety. *Diaphoresis,* or profuse perspiration, accompanies an increased metabolic rate such as occurs in heavy activity or fever.

Diaphoresis occurs with thyrotoxicosis and stimulation of the nervous system with anxiety or pain.

Look for dehydration in the oral mucous membranes. Normally there is none, and the mucous membranes look smooth and moist. Be aware that dark skin may normally look dry and flaky, but this does not necessarily indicate systemic dehydration.

With dehydration mucous membranes look dry, and the lips look parched and cracked. With extreme dryness the skin is fissured, resembling cracks in a desert.

Texture

Normal skin feels smooth and firm, with an even surface.

Hyperthyroidism—The skin feels smoother and softer, like velvet. Hypothyroidism—The skin feels rough, dry, and flaky.

Thickness

The epidermis is uniformly thin over most of the body, although thickened callus areas are normal on palms and soles. A callus is a circumscribed overgrowth of epidermis and is an adaptation to excessive pressure.

Very thin, shiny skin (atrophic) occurs with arterial insufficiency.

Edema

Edema is fluid accumulating in the intercellular spaces and normally is not present. To check for edema, imprint your thumbs firmly against the ankle

Normal Range of Findings	Abnormal Findings

malleolus or the tibia. Normally the skin surface stays smooth when you lift your thumbs. If your pressure leaves a dent in the skin, "pitting" edema is present. Its presence is graded on a four-point scale: from 1+ for mild edema to 4+ for deep pitting edema. This scale is somewhat subjective; outcomes vary among examiners.

Edema is most evident in dependent parts of the body (feet, ankles, and sacral areas) where the skin looks puffy and tight. Edema makes the hair follicles more prominent; thus you note a pigskin or orange-peel look.

Edema masks normal skin color and obscures pathologic conditions such as jaundice or cyanosis because the fluid lies between the surface and the pigmented and vascular layers. It makes dark skin look lighter.

Unilateral edema—Consider a local or peripheral cause.

Bilateral edema or edema that is generalized over the whole body (anasarca) suggests a central problem such as heart or kidney failure.

Mobility and Turgor

Pinch up a large fold of skin on the anterior chest under the clavicle. Mobility is the skin's ease of rising, and turgor is its ability to return to place promptly when released.

Mobility is decreased when edema is present. Poor turgor is evident in severe dehydration or extreme weight loss; the pinched skin recedes slowly or "tents" and stands by itself.

Vascularity or Bruising

Cherry (senile) angiomas are small, smooth, slightly raised, bright red dots that commonly appear on the trunk in adults older than 30 years of age. They normally increase in size and number with aging and are not significant.

Any bruising (contusion) should be consistent with the expected trauma of life. Normally there is no venous dilation or varicosity.

Multiple bruises at different stages of healing and excessive bruises above the knees or elbows raise concern about physical abuse.

Document the presence of any tattoos (a permanent skin design from indelible pigment) on the person's chart. Advise the person that the use of tattoo needles and tattoo parlor equipment of doubtful sterility increases the risk of infection.

Needle marks or tracks from intravenous injection of street drugs may be visible on the antecubital fossae, forearms, or any available vein.

Lesions

Note:
1. Color
2. Elevation: Flat, raised, or pedunculated

Normal Range of Findings	Abnormal Findings

3. Pattern or shape: The grouping or distinctness of each lesion, e.g., annular, grouped, confluent, linear. The pattern may be characteristic of a certain disease.
4. Size in centimeters: Use a ruler to measure. Avoid descriptions such as "quarter size" or "pea size."
5. Location and distribution on body. Is it generalized or localized to area of a specific irritant (around jewelry, watchband, around eyes)?
6. Any exudate? Note its color or odor.

Wear a glove if you anticipate contact with blood, mucosa, any body fluid, or an open skin lesion.

Lesions are traumatic or pathologic changes in previously normal structures. When a lesion develops on previously unaltered skin, it is **primary.** However, when a lesion changes over time or because of a factor such as scratching or infection, it is **secondary.**

Study Table 5.2 on p. 48 for pattern and Tables 5.3 and 5.4 on pp. 49-52 for the characteristics of primary and secondary skin lesions.

Inspect and Palpate the Hair

Color

Hair color comes from melanin production and may vary from pale blonde to total black. Graying begins as early as the 30s as a result of genetic factors.

Texture

Scalp hair may be fine or thick and look straight, curly, or kinky. It should look shiny.

Note dull, coarse, or brittle scalp hair.

Lesions

The scalp should be clean and free of any lesions or pest inhabitants. Many people normally have seborrhea (dandruff), which is indicated by loose white flakes.

Distinguish dandruff from nits (eggs) of lice, which are oval, adhere to the hair shaft, and cause intense itching.

Inspect and Palpate the Nails

Shape and Contour

The nail surface is normally slightly curved or flat, and the posterior and lateral nail folds are smooth and rounded. Nail edges are smooth, rounded, and clean, suggesting adequate self-care.

Spoon nails (concave curves) may occur with iron-deficiency anemia.
Paronychia (inflammation of base of nail) occurs with trauma or infection.

Normal Range of Findings	Abnormal Findings
	Jagged nails, nails bitten to the quick, or traumatized nail folds from chronic nervous picking suggest nervous habits.
	Chronically dirty nails suggest poor self-care or occupations in which it is impossible to keep them clean.
View the index finger at its profile and note the angle of the nail base; it should be about 160 degrees. The nail base is firm to palpation. Curved nails with a convex profile are a variation of normal. They may look like clubbed nails, but notice that the angle between nail base and nail is normal (i.e., 160 degrees or less).	Clubbing of nails occurs with congenital, cyanotic heart disease; emphysema; and chronic bronchitis. In early clubbing the angle straightens out to 180 degrees, and the nail base feels spongy to palpation (see Fig. 13.13, p. 211, in Jarvis: *Physical Examination and Health Assessment,* 8th ed.).
Consistency	
The nail surface is smooth and regular, not brittle or splitting.	Pits, transverse grooves, or lines may indicate a nutrient deficiency or accompany acute illness with disturbed nail growth.
Nail thickness is uniform.	Nails are thickened, ridged, with arterial insufficiency.
The nail adheres firmly to the nail bed, and the nail base is firm to palpation.	A spongy nail base accompanies clubbing.
Color	
The translucent nail plate shows a pink nail bed underneath.	Cyanosis or marked pallor.
Dark-skinned people may have brown-black pigmented areas or linear bands or streaks along the nail edge. Many people normally have white hairline linear markings from trauma or picking at the cuticle. Note any abnormal markings in the nail beds.	Brown linear streaks are abnormal in light-skinned people and may indicate melanoma.
Capillary Refill. Depress the nail edge to blanch and then release, noting the return of color. Normally color return is instant or within a few seconds in a cold environment. This indicates the status of the peripheral circulation. A sluggish color return takes longer than 1 or 2 seconds.	Splinter hemorrhages occur with subacute bacterial endocarditis; transverse ridges, or Beau's lines, occur with trauma.
	Cyanotic nail beds or sluggish color return—Consider cardiovascular or respiratory dysfunction.

Normal Range of Findings	Abnormal Findings

DEVELOPMENTAL COMPETENCE

Infants

General Pigmentation. Black newborns initially have lighter-toned skin than their parents. Their full melanotic color is evident in the nail beds and scrotal folds.

The **Mongolian spot** is a common variation of hyperpigmentation in black, Native American, Hispanic, and Asian newborns as a result of deep dermal melanocytes. It is a blue-black–to-purple macular area usually found at the sacrum or buttocks. It gradually fades during the first year of life.

Bruising is a common soft tissue injury that follows a rapid, traumatic, or breech birth.

Multiple bruises in various stages of healing, or pattern injury, that do not match history, suggest physical abuse.

Adolescents

The increase in sebaceous gland activity creates increased oiliness and acne.

The Pregnant Female

Striae are jagged linear "stretch marks" of silver to pink that appear during the 2nd trimester on the abdomen, breasts, and sometimes on the thighs. They occur in one-half of all pregnancies and fade after delivery but do not disappear. On the abdomen the **linea nigra** appears as a brownish-black line down the midline.

Chloasma is an irregular brown patch of hyperpigmentation on the face. It may occur with pregnancy or in women taking oral contraceptive pills. Chloasma disappears after delivery or cessation of pill use.

Vascular spiders occur in two-thirds of pregnancies in white women but less often in black women. These lesions have tiny red centers with radiating branches and occur on the face, neck, upper chest, and arms.

The Aging Adult

Skin Color and Pigmentation. **Senile lentigines** are commonly called *liver spots* and are small, flat, brown macules that appear after extensive sun

Normal Range of Findings	Abnormal Findings

exposure on the forearms and dorsa of the hands. They are not malignant and require no treatment.

Moisture. Dry skin (xerosis) is common. The skin itches and appears flaky and loose.

Texture. Acrochordons, or "skin tags," are overgrowths of normal skin that form a stalk and occur frequently on the eyelids, cheeks, neck, axillae, and trunk.

Thickness. With aging the skin looks as thin as parchment, and subcutaneous fat diminishes. Thinner skin is evident over the dorsa of the hands, forearms, lower legs, feet, and bony prominences.

Aging skin increases risk for pressure injuries (see Table 5.5, pp. 53-54).

Mobility and Turgor. Turgor is decreased (less elasticity), and the skin recedes slowly or "tents" and stands by itself.

Hair. Hair growth decreases, and the amount decreases in the axillae and pubic areas. After menopause white women may develop bristly hairs on the chin or upper lip as a result of unopposed androgens.

In men, coarse terminal hairs develop in the ears, nose, and eyebrows, although the beard is unchanged. Male pattern balding, or **alopecia,** is a genetic trait. It is usually a gradual receding of the anterior hairline in a symmetric W shape.

In men and women scalp hair gradually turns gray because of a decrease in melanocyte function.

Nails. Nail growth rate decreases, and local injuries in the nail matrix may produce longitudinal ridges. The surface may be brittle or peeling and sometimes is yellowed. Toenails also are thickened and may grow misshapen, almost grotesque. The thickening can be a process of aging or is caused by chronic peripheral vascular disease.

Fungal infections are common in aging, with thickened, crumbling toenails and erythematous scaling on contiguous skin surfaces.

For more information on assessment of skin, hair, and nails, see Jarvis: *Physical Examination and Health Assessment,* 8th ed., pp. 197-244.

HEALTH PROMOTION AND PATIENT TEACHING

Teach all adults to examine their skin once a month, using the ABCDE rule to raise warning signals of any suspicious lesions. Use a well-lit room that has a full-length mirror. It helps to have a small handheld mirror. Ask a relative to search skin areas difficult to see (e.g., behind ears, back of neck, back). Follow the sequence outlined in the following list and report any suspicious lesions promptly to a physician or nurse.

1. Undress completely. Check forearms, palms, space between fingers. Turn over hands and study the backs.
2. Face mirror, bend arms at elbows. Study arms in mirror.
3. Face mirror and study entire body front. Start at face and neck, working over torso and down to lower legs.
4. Pivot to have right side facing mirror. Study sides of upper arms, working down to ankles. Repeat with left side.
5. With back to mirror, study buttocks, thighs, lower legs.
6. Use handheld mirror to study upper back.
7. Use handheld mirror to study scalp, lifting the hair. A blow-dryer on a cool setting helps to lift hair.
8. Sit on chair or bed. Study insides of each leg and soles of feet. Use small mirror to help.

Summary Checklist: Skin, Hair, and Nails

For a PDA-downloadable version go to http://evolve.elsevier.com/Jarvis.

1. **Inspect the skin:**
   Color
   General pigmentation
   Areas of hypopigmentation or hyperpigmentation
   Abnormal color changes
2. **Palpate the skin:**
   Temperature
   Moisture
   Texture
   Thickness
   Edema
   Mobility and turgor
   Vascularity or bruising
3. **Note any lesions:**
   Color
   Shape and configuration
   Size
   Location and distribution on body
4. **Inspect and palpate the hair:**
   Texture
   Distribution
   Any scalp lesions
5. **Inspect and palpate the nails:**
   Shape and contour
   Consistency
   Color
6. **Teach skin self-examination**

DOCUMENTATION

Sample Charting

SUBJECTIVE

No history of skin disease; no present change in pigmentation or in nevi; no pruritus, bruising, rash, or lesions. Taking no medications. No work-related skin hazards. Uses SPF 30 sun-block cream when outdoors.

OBJECTIVE

Skin: Color tan-pink, even pigmentation, with no suspicious nevi. Warm to touch, dry, smooth, and even. Turgor good, no lesions.
Hair: Even distribution, thick texture, no lesions or pest inhabitants.
Nails: No clubbing or deformities. Nail beds pink with prompt capillary refill.

ASSESSMENT

Warm, dry, intact skin.

ABNORMAL FINDINGS

TABLE 5.1	Color Changes in Light and Dark Skin	
Etiology	Light Skin	Dark Skin
Pallor		
Anemia—Decreased hematocrit Shock—Decreased perfusion, vasoconstriction	Generalized pallor	Brown skin appears yellow-brown, dull; black skin appears ashen gray, dull; skin loses its healthy glow Check areas with least pigmentation such as conjunctivae, mucous membranes
Local arterial insufficiency	Marked localized pallor (e.g., lower extremities, especially when elevated)	Ashen gray, dull; cool to palpation
Albinism—Total absence of pigment melanin throughout the integument	Whitish pink	Tan, cream, white
Vitiligo—Patchy depigmentation from destruction of melanocytes	Patchy milky white spots, often symmetric bilaterally	Same
Cyanosis		
Increased amount of unoxygenated hemoglobin Central—Chronic heart and lung disease cause arterial desaturation Peripheral—Exposure to cold, anxiety	Dusky blue Nail beds dusky	Dark but dull, lifeless Only severe cyanosis is apparent in skin—check conjunctivae, oral mucosa, nail beds
Erythema		
Hyperemia—Increased blood in engorged arterioles: inflammation, fever, alcohol intake, blushing	Red, bright pink	Purplish tinge but difficult to see; palpate for increased warmth with inflammation, for taut skin and hardening of deep tissues
Polycythemia—Increased red blood cells, capillary stasis	Ruddy blue in face, oral mucosa, conjunctivae, hands and feet	Well-concealed by pigment Check for redness in lips

Continued

TABLE 5.1	Color Changes in Light and Dark Skin—cont'd	
Etiology	Light Skin	Dark Skin
Carbon monoxide poisoning	Bright cherry red in face and upper torso	Cherry red color in nail beds, lips, and oral mucosa
Venous stasis—Decreased blood flow from area, engorged venules	Dusky rubor of dependent extremities; a prelude to necrosis with pressure sores	Easily masked; use palpation for warmth of edema
Jaundice		
Increased serum bilirubin due to liver inflammation or hemolytic disease, such as after severe burns or some infections	Yellow in sclerae, hard palate, mucous membranes, then over skin	Check sclera for yellow near limbus; do not mistake normal yellowish fatty deposits in the periphery under the eyelids for jaundice Jaundice best noted in junction of hard and soft palate and also in palms
Carotenemia—Increased serum carotene from ingestion of large amounts of carotene-rich foods	Yellow-orange in forehead, palms and soles, and nasolabial folds; but no yellowing in sclerae or mucous membranes	Yellow-orange tinge in palms and soles
Uremia—Renal failure causes retained urochrome pigments in the blood	Orange-green or gray overlying pallor of anemia; may also have ecchymoses and purpura	Easily masked by dark skin; rely on laboratory and clinical findings
Brown-Tan		
Addison's disease—Cortisol deficiency stimulates increased melanin production	Bronzed appearance, an "eternal tan"; most apparent around nipples, perineum, genitalia, and pressure points (inner thighs, buttocks, elbows, axillae)	Easily masked by dark skin; rely on laboratory and clinical findings
Café-au-lait spots—Due to increased melanin pigment in basal cell layer	Tan to light brown, irregularly shaped, oval patches with well-defined borders	

TABLE 5.2	Common Shapes of Skin Lesions

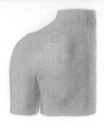 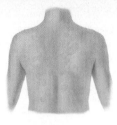 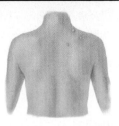

ANNULAR: Circular lesions that begin in center and spread to periphery (e.g., ringworm, tinea versicolor, pityriasis rosea)

CONFLUENT: Lesions that run together (e.g., urticaria)

DISCRETE: Distinct, individual lesions that remain separate

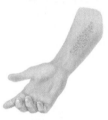 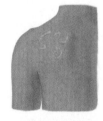 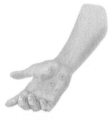

GROUPED: Clusters of lesions (e.g., vesicles of contact dermatitis)

GYRATE: Twisted, coiled spiral, or snakelike lesions

IRIS or TARGET: Lesions that resemble iris of eye, concentric rings of lesions

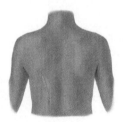 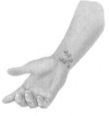 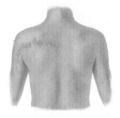

LINEAR: Lesions take form of a scratch, streak, line, or stripe

POLYCYCLIC: Annular lesions that grow together

ZOSTERIFORM: Lesions take linear arrangement along nerve route (e.g., herpes zoster)

TABLE 5.3 Primary Skin Lesions[a]

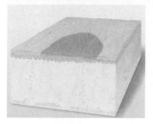

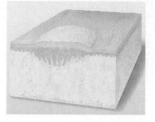

MACULE: Solely a color change, flat and circumscribed, <1 cm. Examples: Freckle, flat nevus, petechia, measles, scarlet fever

PATCH: Macule larger than 1 cm. Examples: Mongolian spot, vitiligo, café-au-lait spot, chloasma, measles rash

PAPULE: Something you can palpate, i.e., solid, elevated, circumscribed lesion <1 cm in diameter. Examples: Elevated nevus (mole), lichen planus, molluscum, wart (verruca)

PLAQUE: Papules coalesce wider than 1 cm to form a plateaulike, disc-shaped lesion. Examples: Psoriasis, lichen planus

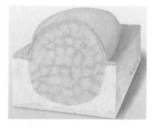

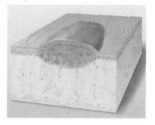

NODULE: Solid, elevated, hard or soft lesion larger than 1 cm; may extend deeper into dermis than papule. Examples: Xanthoma, fibroma, intradermal nevus

TUMOR: Lesion larger than a few centimeters in diameter, firm or soft, deeper into dermis; may be benign or malignant. Examples: Lipoma, hemangioma

WHEAL: Superficial, raised, transient, and erythematous lesion; has slightly irregular shape caused by edema (fluid held diffusely in the tissues). Examples: Mosquito bite, allergic reaction, dermographism

URTICARIA (HIVES): Wheals coalesce to form extensive reaction; intensely pruritic

[a]The immediate result of a specific causative factor; primary lesions develop on previously unaltered skin.

Continued

TABLE 5.3	Primary Skin Lesions^a—cont'd

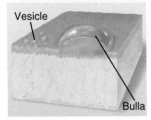

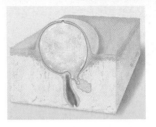

VESICLE: Elevated cavity containing free clear fluid, up to 1 cm. Examples: Herpes simplex, early varicella (chickenpox), herpes zoster (shingles), contact dermatitis

BULLA: Larger than 1 cm in diameter; usually single chambered (unilocular); superficial in epidermis; thin walled, so it ruptures easily. Examples: Friction blister, pemphigus, burns, contact dermatitis

PUSTULE: Turbid fluid (pus) in cavity; circumscribed and elevated. Examples: Impetigo, acne

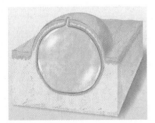

CYST: Encapsulated, fluid-filled cavity in dermis or subcutaneous layer that tensely elevates skin. Examples: Sebaceous cyst, wen

Images © Pat Thomas, 2010.

TABLE 5.4	Secondary Skin Lesions[a]

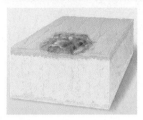

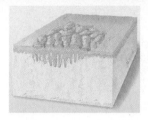

CRUST: Thickened, dried-out exudate left when vesicles or pustules burst or dry up. Color can be red-brown, honey, or yellow, depending on the fluid's ingredients (blood, serum, pus). Examples: Impetigo (dry, honey colored), weeping eczematous dermatitis, scab following abrasion

SCALE: Compact, desiccated flakes of skin, dry or greasy, silvery or white, from shedding of dead excess keratin cells. Examples: Following drug reaction (laminated sheets), psoriasis (silver, micalike), seborrheic dermatitis (yellow, greasy), eczema, (large, adherent, laminated), dry skin

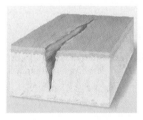

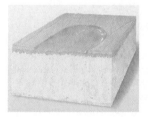

FISSURE: Linear crack with abrupt edges, extending into dermis; dry or moist. Examples: Cheilosis at corners of mouth due to excess moisture; athlete's foot

EROSION: Scooped-out but shallow depression; superficial lesion, epidermis is lost, and the lesion is moist but there is no bleeding; heals without scar because erosion does not extend into dermis.

[a]Resulting from a change in a primary lesion because of the passage of time; an evolutionary change.
NOTE: Combinations of primary and secondary lesions may coexist in the same person. Such combined designations may be termed *papulosquamous*, *maculopapular*, *vesiculopustular*, or *papulovesicular*.

Continued

TABLE 5.4	Secondary Skin Lesions[a]—cont'd

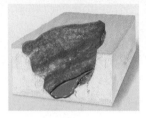

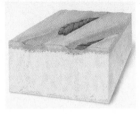

ULCER: Deeper depression, extending into dermis, irregularly shaped. It may bleed and leaves scar when it heals. Examples: Stasis ulcer, pressure sore, chancre

EXCORIATION: Self-inflicted abrasion; superficial and sometimes crusted. Examples: Scratches from intense itching from insect bite, scabies, dermatitis, varicella

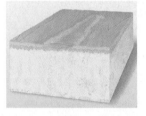

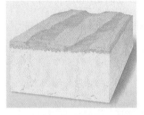

SCAR: After a skin lesion is repaired, normal tissue is lost and replaced with connective tissue (collagen); a permanent fibrotic change. Examples: Healed area of surgery or injury, acne

ATROPHIC SCAR: Resulting skin level depressed with loss of tissue; thinning of the epidermis. Example: Striae

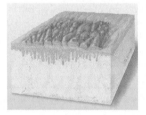

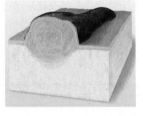

LICHENIFICATION: Prolonged intense scratching eventually thickens the skin and produces tightly packed sets of papules: looks like surface of moss (or lichen).

KELOID: Hypertrophic scar; resulting skin level is elevated by excess scar tissue, which is invasive beyond the site of original injury; may increase long after healing occurs; looks smooth, rubbery, "clawlike"; higher incidence among blacks.

Images © Pat Thomas, 2010.

TABLE 5.5	Pressure Injury (PI) (Pressure Ulcer, Decubitus Ulcer)

PIs appear on the skin over a bony prominence when circulation is impaired. This occurs when confined to bed or immobilized. Immobilization slows delivery of blood-carrying oxygen and nutrients to the skin, and it slows venous drainage carrying metabolic wastes away from the skin. This results in ischemia and cell death. Common sites for pressure ulcers are on the back (heel, ischium, sacrum, elbow, scapula, vertebra) or the side (ankle, knee, hip, rib, shoulder).

Risk factors for PIs include impaired mobility; thin fragile skin of aging; decreased sensory perception (thus unable to respond to pain accompanying prolonged pressure); impaired level of consciousness (also unable to respond); moisture from urine or stool incontinence, excessive perspiration, or wound drainage; shearing injury (being pulled down or across in bed); poor nutrition; and infection. Knowledge of risk factors and prevention of pressure ulcers are far more easily accomplished than is treatment of existing ulcers. However, once pressure ulcers occur, they are assessed by stage, depending on the pressure ulcer depth (NPUAP, 2016):

Stage I—Nonblanchable Erythema

Intact skin appears red but unbroken. Localized redness in light skin blanches (turns light with fingertip pressure). Dark skin appears darker but does not blanch.

Stage II—Partial-Thickness Skin Loss

Partial-thickness skin erosion with loss of epidermis or also the dermis. Superficial ulcer looks shallow, like an abrasion or open blister with a red-pink wound bed.

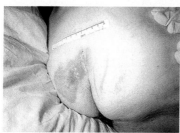

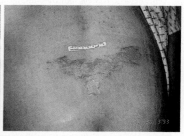

Continued

TABLE 5.5	Pressure Injury (PI) (Pressure Ulcer, Decubitus Ulcer)—cont'd

Stage III—Full-Thickness Skin Loss

Full-thickness skin loss extending into the subcutaneous tissue and resembling a crater. May see subcutaneous fat, but not muscle, bone, or tendon.

Stage IV—Full-Thickness Skin/Tissue Loss

Full-thickness PI involves all skin layers and extends into supporting tissue. Exposes muscle, tendon, or bone, and may show slough (stringy matter attached to wound bed) or eschar (black or brown necrotic tissue).

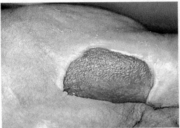 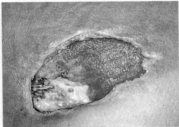

Once Stage III or IV ulcers occur, wound size must be measured weekly to provide quantifiable data for wound healing. Use disposable rulers with millimeter and centimeter markings, and measure greatest overall wound length and width.

Deep Tissue Pressure Injury (DTPI)

Localized, nonblanchable color change to deep red, maroon, or purple in intact or nonintact skin. Dark skin appears darker but does not blanch. Or, epidermis may separate, revealing dark wound or blood-filled blister (NPUAP, 2016). Preceded by pain and temperature change. Begins in the muscle closest to the bone, in older adults and in those with a lower BMI, commonly on skin over coccyx, sacrum, buttocks, heels (Preston et al., 2017).

PI Caused by Medical Device

Skin or mucosa has PI that looks like pattern or shape of medical device (e.g., IV hub, endotracheal tube, cervical collar, anti-thromboembolism stocking) (Delmore & Ayello, 2017).

See Illustration Credits for source information.

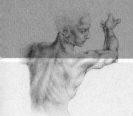

Head, Face, Neck, and Regional Lymphatics

ANATOMY

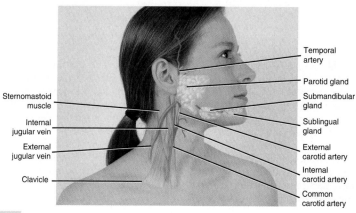

Temporal artery
Parotid gland
Submandibular gland
Sublingual gland
External carotid artery
Internal carotid artery
Common carotid artery

Sternomastoid muscle
Internal jugular vein
External jugular vein
Clavicle

6.1

Facial structures are symmetric; the eyebrows, eyes, ears, nose, and mouth appear about the same on both sides. The palpebral fissures—the openings between the eyelids—are equal bilaterally. The nasolabial folds—the creases extending from the nose to each corner of the mouth—should look symmetric. Facial sensations of pain or touch are mediated by the three sensory branches of cranial nerve V, the trigeminal nerve. The facial expressions are formed by the muscles mediated by cranial nerve VII, the facial nerve.

Two pairs of salivary glands are accessible to examination on the face (Fig. 6.1). The parotid glands are in the cheeks over the mandible, anterior to and below the ear. They are the largest of the salivary glands but normally are not palpable. The submandibular glands are beneath the mandible at the angle of the jaw. A third pair, the sublingual glands, lies in the floor of the mouth. The temporal artery lies superior to the temporalis muscle, and its pulsation is palpable anterior to the ear.

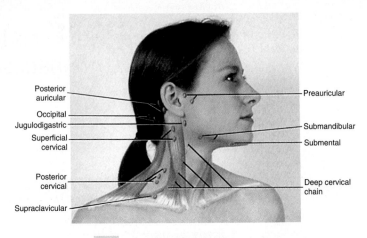

Posterior auricular
Occipital
Jugulodigastric
Superficial cervical
Posterior cervical
Supraclavicular

Preauricular
Submandibular
Submental
Deep cervical chain

6.2 Lymph nodes of the head and neck.

The head and neck have a rich supply of lymph nodes (Fig. 6.2). The nodes are small oval clusters of lymphatic tissue. They filter the lymph and engulf pathogens, thereby preventing potentially harmful substances from entering the circulation.

The neck contains many structures lying in close proximity (Fig. 6.3). The major neck muscles are the **sternomastoid** and also the **trapezius** on the upper back. The carotid artery and internal jugular vein lie beneath the sternomastoid muscle. (see assessment of the neck vessels in Chapter 12.) The **thyroid gland** straddles the trachea, and its two lobes each curve posteriorly between the trachea and sternomastoid muscle. This highly vascular endocrine gland secretes thyroid hormones for cellular metabolism.

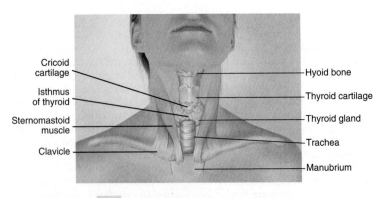

Cricoid cartilage
Isthmus of thyroid
Sternomastoid muscle
Clavicle

Hyoid bone
Thyroid cartilage
Thyroid gland
Trachea
Manubrium

6.3 Landmarks and structures in the neck.

SUBJECTIVE DATA

1. Headache
2. Head injury
3. Dizziness
4. Neck pain
5. Limitation of motion
6. Lumps or swelling

OBJECTIVE DATA

Normal Range of Findings	Abnormal Findings

The Head

Inspect and Palpate the Skull

Normocephalic describes a round, symmetric skull appropriately related to body size.

Microcephaly—Abnormally small head.

The skull normally feels symmetric and smooth. The cranial bones with normal protrusions are the forehead, the lateral edge of each parietal bone, the occipital bone, and the mastoid process behind each ear. There is no tenderness to palpation.

Macrocephaly—Abnormally large head (e.g., hydrocephaly and acromegaly).

Lumps, depressions, or abnormal protrusions.

Palpate the temporal artery above the zygomatic (cheek) bone between the eye and the top of the ear.

Tenderness.

Palpate the temporomandibular joints located anterior to each ear as the person opens the mouth, and note normally smooth movement with no limitation or tenderness.

Crepitation, limited range of motion, or tenderness.

Inspect the Face

Note the facial expression and its appropriateness to behavior or reported mood. Anxiety is common in hospitalized or ill persons.

Hostility or aggression. Tense, rigid muscles may indicate anxiety or pain; a flat affect may indicate depression.

Note symmetry of eyebrows, palpebral fissures, nasolabial folds, and sides of the mouth. Note any abnormal facial structures (coarse facial features, exophthalmos, changes in skin color or pigmentation) or any abnormal swelling. Also note any involuntary movements (tics) in the facial muscles. Normally there are none.

Marked asymmetry shows with central brain lesion (e.g., stroke) or with peripheral cranial nerve VII damage (e.g., Bell palsy). (See Table 14.5, p. 272, in Jarvis: *Physical Examination and Health Assessment*, 8th ed.)

Edema in the face is noted first around the eyes (periorbital) and the cheeks, where the subcutaneous tissue is relatively loose.

Normal Range of Findings	Abnormal Findings
	Note grinding of jaws, tics or fasciculations, or excessive blinking.

The Neck

Inspect and Palpate the Neck

Symmetry. Head position is in the midline; accessory neck muscles are symmetric.

Head tilt occurs with muscle spasm. Head and neck rigidity occurs with arthritis.

Range of Motion. Ask the person to touch the chin to the chest, turn the head to the right and left, try to touch each ear to the shoulder (without elevating shoulders), and extend the head backward. When the neck is supple, motion is smooth and controlled.

Note any limitation of movement. Note pain at any particular movement.

Note ratchety movement or limitation of movement, as with cervical arthritis or inflammation of neck muscles. With arthritis the neck is rigid, and the person turns at the shoulders rather than the neck.

Lymph Nodes. Using a gentle circular motion of your finger pads and beginning with the preauricular lymph nodes in front of the ear, palpate the 10 groups of lymph nodes in a routine order. Be systematic and thorough. Use gentle pressure because strong pressure could push the nodes into the neck muscles. It is usually most efficient to palpate with both hands, comparing the two sides for the symmetry.

Lymphadenopathy is palpable enlargement of the lymph nodes (>1 cm) from infection, allergy, or neoplasm.

The following are commonly associated with lymphadenopathy but are not definitive in all circumstances:

If any nodes are palpable, note their location, size, shape, delimitation (discrete or matted together), mobility, consistency, and tenderness. Cervical nodes often are palpable in healthy people, although palpability decreases with age. Normal nodes feel movable, discrete, soft, and nontender.

- Acute infection—Nodes are bilateral, enlarged, warm, tender, and firm but freely movable.

- Chronic inflammation, e.g., in tuberculosis the nodes are clumped.
- Cancerous nodes are hard, enlarged, unilateral, nontender, and fixed.
- Nodes in persons with HIV infection are enlarged, firm, nontender, and mobile. Occipital lymphadenopathy is common.

If nodes are enlarged or tender, check the area they drain for the source of the problem. Look proximal (upstream) to the location of the node, e.g., the nodes in the upper cervical or submandibular area often relate to inflammation or a neoplasm in the head and neck. Follow up on or refer your findings. An enlarged lymph node deserves prompt attention, particularly when you cannot find the source of the problem.

- A single enlarged, nontender, hard left supraclavicular node may indicate a neoplasm in the thorax or abdomen.
- Painless, rubbery, discrete nodes that appear gradually occur with Hodgkin lymphoma.

Normal Range of Findings	Abnormal Findings

Thyroid Gland. Position a standing lamp to shine tangentially across the neck to highlight any possible swelling. Supply the person with a glass of water and first inspect the neck as the person takes a sip and swallows. Thyroid tissue moves up with a swallow.

To palpate the thyroid, move behind the person (Fig. 6.4). Ask him or her to sit up very straight and then bend the head slightly forward and to the right. This relaxes the neck muscles on the right side. Use the fingers of your left hand to push the trachea slightly to the right.

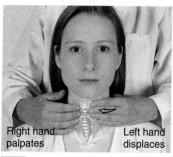

Right hand palpates   Left hand displaces

6.4

Curve your right fingers between the trachea and the sternomastoid muscle, retracting it slightly, and ask the person to take a sip of water. The thyroid moves up under your fingers with the trachea and larynx as the person swallows. Reverse the procedure for the left side.

Usually you cannot palpate a normal adult thyroid. If the person has a long, thin neck, you sometimes can feel the thyroid isthmus over the tracheal rings. The lateral lobes usually are not palpable; check them for enlargement, consistency, symmetry, and the presence of nodules.

Abnormalities include enlarged lobes that are easily palpated before swallowing or that are tender to palpation or the presence of nodules or lumps (see Table 14.3, p. 269, in Jarvis: *Physical Examination and Health Assessment,* 8th ed.).

Normal Range of Findings	Abnormal Findings

 DEVELOPMENTAL COMPETENCE

Infants and Children. An infant's head size is measured with measuring tape at each visit up to age 2. (Measurement of head circumference is presented in detail in Chapter 4.)

Gently palpate the skull and fontanels while the infant is calm and in a somewhat sitting position (crying, lying down, or vomiting may cause the anterior fontanel to look full and bulging). The skull should feel smooth and fused except at the fontanels. The fontanels feel firm, slightly concave, and well defined against the edges of the cranial bones.

You may see slight arterial pulsations in the anterior fontanel.

The posterior fontanel may not be palpable at birth. If it is, it measures 1 cm and closes by age 1 to 2 months. The anterior fontanel may be small at birth and enlarge to 2.5 cm × 2.5 cm. A large diameter of 4 to 5 cm occasionally may be normal at younger than 6 months.

The anterior fontanel closes between 9 months and 2 years. Early closure may be insignificant if head growth proceeds normally.

During infancy, cervical lymph nodes normally are not palpable, but a child's lymph nodes are. They feel more prominent than an adult's until puberty, when lymphoid tissue begins to atrophy. Palpable nodes less than 3 mm are normal. They may be up to 1 cm in size in the cervical and inguinal areas but are discrete, move easily, and are nontender. Children have a higher incidence of infection; so you expect

Microcephaly—Head circumference below norms for age.

Macrocephaly—Head that is enlarged for age or rapidly increasing in size. This may be caused by hydrocephalus (increased cerebrospinal fluid).

A true tense or bulging fontanel occurs with acute increased intracranial pressure.

Depressed and sunken fontanels occur with dehydration or malnutrition.

Marked pulsations occur with increased intracranial pressure.

Delayed closure or larger-than-normal fontanels occur with hydrocephalus, Down syndrome, hypothyroidism, or rickets.

A small fontanel is a sign of microcephaly, as is early closure.

Cervical nodes larger than 1 cm are considered enlarged.

Thyroglossal duct cyst—Cystic lymph node high up in the midline that is freely movable and that rises up during swallowing.

Normal Range of Findings	Abnormal Findings
a greater incidence of inflammatory adenopathy. There should be no other mass in the neck.	Supraclavicular nodes enlarge with Hodgkin disease.

The Pregnant Woman. The thyroid gland normally may be palpable during pregnancy as a result of hyperplasia of the tissue and increased vascularity.

The Aging Adult. In some aging adults a mild rhythmic tremor of the head is normal. *Senile tremors* are benign and include head nodding (as if saying yes or no) and tongue protrusion.

If some teeth have been lost, the lower face looks unusually small, with the mouth sunken in.

The neck may show an increased cervical concave curve when the head and jaw are extended forward to compensate for kyphosis of the spine. During the examination direct the older adult to perform range of motion slowly; he or she may experience dizziness with side movements.

For more information on assessment of the head and neck, see Jarvis: *Physical Examination and Health Assessment,* 8th ed., pp. 245-274.

Summary Checklist: Head, Face, and Neck

1. **Inspect and palpate the skull:**
   General size and contour
   Note any deformities, lumps, tenderness
   Palpate temporal artery and temporomandibular joint
2. **Inspect the face:**
   Facial expression
   Symmetry of movement (cranial nerve VII)
   Any involuntary movements, edema, lesions
3. **Inspect and palpate the neck:**
   Active range of motion
   Enlargement of lymph nodes or thyroid gland

HEALTH PROMOTION AND PATIENT TEACHING

(To the parents of a newborn.) *"Because your baby sleeps flat on the back, I would like to teach you about tummy time during the day; place the baby on his or her tummy while awake and supervised."* A newborn can be prone on the parent's lap 2 to 3 times a day for a few minutes, with a gradual increase to 20 minutes a day on the floor for a 3- to 4-month-old.

(To young athletes and parents of athletes.) *"We want you to stay safe in your sport, and most athletes and parents do not know the signs of concussion. A concussion is a direct blow to the head, causing the brain inside to rattle back and forth on its attachments. Serious signs of concussion are forgetfulness of recent events, loss of consciousness, and mental cloudiness. Other signs are headache, nausea and vomiting, loss of balance, and blurred vision. Later signs include difficulty in concentrating, poor short-term memory, slow reaction time, and irritability"* (Jamault & Duff, 2013).

DOCUMENTATION

Sample Charting

SUBJECTIVE

Denies any unusually frequent or severe headache; no history of head injury, dizziness, or syncope; no neck pain, limitation of motion, lumps, or swelling.

OBJECTIVE

Head: Normocephalic, no lumps, no lesions, no tenderness, no trauma.
Face: Symmetric, no drooping, no weakness, no involuntary movements.
Neck: Supple with full ROM, no pain. Symmetric, no cervical lymphadenopathy or masses. Trachea midline, thyroid not palpable. No bruits.

ASSESSMENT

Normocephalic, atraumatic, and symmetric head and neck.

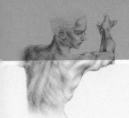

CHAPTER 7

Eyes

ANATOMY

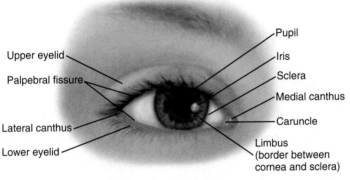

Upper eyelid

Palpebral fissure

Lateral canthus

Lower eyelid

Pupil

Iris

Sclera

Medial canthus

Caruncle

Limbus
(border between
cornea and sclera)

7.1 External eye structures. (© Pat Thomas, 2006.)

The eye is the sensory organ of vision. The eyelids protect the eye from injury, strong light, and dust (Fig. 7.1). The **palpebral fissure** is the open space between the eyelids.

The exposed part of the eye has a transparent protective covering, the **conjunctiva**. The *palpebral* conjunctiva lines the lids and is clear, with many small blood vessels. It forms a deep recess and then folds back over the eye. The *bulbar* conjunctiva overlays the eyeball, with the white sclera showing

through. At the limbus the conjunctiva merges with the cornea. The **cornea** covers and protects the iris and pupil.

The eye is a sphere composed of three concentric coats: (1) the outer fibrous **sclera,** (2) the middle vascular **choroid,** and (3) the inner nervous **retina** (Fig. 7.2). Inside the retina is the transparent vitreous body.

The retina is the visual receptive layer of the eye in which light waves are changed into nerve impulses. The

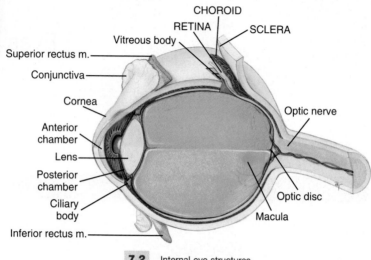

7.2 Internal eye structures.

ocular fundus is the area of the retina visible through the ophthalmoscope (Fig. 7.3).

The **optic disc** is the area in which fibers from the retina converge to form the optic nerve. The **macula** is the area of sharpest vision.

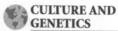
CULTURE AND GENETICS

Cataracts are a leading cause of blindness worldwide, and it is estimated that 80% of the cases of this visual impairment are preventable or curable with surgery (Mundy, Nichols, &

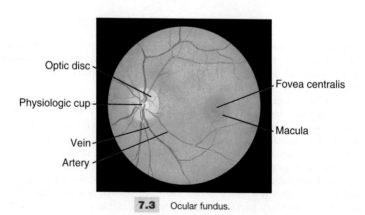

7.3 Ocular fundus.

Londsey, 2016). In the United States, African-American men and women were more likely to have cataracts in every age category (Kaiser, Friedman, & Pineda, 2014). Cataract surgery is cost-effective in alleviating a preventable cause of visual impairment, and it may help relieve the burden of poverty by returning people to the work force and increasing social mobility.

Glaucoma prevalence increases with advancing age; in the United States, African Americans are 3 to 6 times more likely to develop the condition than are whites. Primary open-angle glaucoma is the leading cause of blindness in African Americans and Hispanics (Kaiser, Friedman, & Pineda, 2014; Gupta & Chen, 2016).

Age-related macular degeneration shows changes in 19.7% of U.S. adults over 75 years; it is more prevalent in whites. Additional risk factors include positive family history, cigarette smoking, hyperopia, light iris color, hypertension, hypercholesterolemia, and female gender (Kaiser, Friedman, & Pineda, 2014).

Visual impairment (VI) is not being able to see letters on the eye chart at line 20/50 or below. In the United States, the number of people with VI and blindness is expected to double because of the aging population and shifting demographics (Varma et al., 2016). In 2015 the highest numbers were found in whites, women, and older adults, and that will be true in 2050. In 2015 African Americans were the minority group with the highest prevalence of VI and blindness; this will shift to Hispanic people in 2050 as they are the fastest-growing minority group.

SUBJECTIVE DATA

1. Vision difficulty (decreased acuity, blurring, blind spots)
2. Pain
3. Strabismus, diplopia
4. Redness, swelling
5. Watering, discharge
6. Past history of ocular problems
7. Glaucoma
8. Use of glasses or contact lenses
9. Patient-centered care (vision last tested, method of care for contacts or glasses, efforts to protect eyes)

OBJECTIVE DATA

EQUIPMENT NEEDED

Snellen eye chart
Handheld visual screener
Opaque card or occluder

Penlight
Ophthalmoscope

Normal Range of Findings	Abnormal Findings

Test Central Visual Acuity

Snellen Eye Chart

Position the person on a mark exactly 20 feet from the chart. Leave glasses or contact lenses in place. Shield one eye at a time during the test. Ask the person to read through the chart to the smallest line of letters possible.

Record the result using the numeric fraction at the end of the last successful line read. Indicate whether any letters were missed and whether corrective lenses were worn (e.g., "Right eye 20/30—1, with glasses").

Normal visual acuity is 20/20. The top number (numerator) indicates the distance the person is standing from the chart; the denominator gives the distance at which a normal eye can read a particular line.

Near Vision

For people older than 40 years of age or for those who report increasing difficulty reading, test near vision using a handheld vision screener with various sizes of print (e.g., a Jaeger card). Hold the card in good light about 35 cm (14 inches) from the eye. Test each eye separately with glasses on. A normal result is "14/14" in each eye read without hesitancy and without moving the card closer or farther away.

Test Visual Fields

Confrontation Test

Position yourself at eye level with the patient and about 2 feet away. Direct him or her to cover one eye with an opaque card and look straight at you with the other eye. Hold your finger as a target midline between you and the other person and slowly advance it in from the periphery in several directions (upward, downward, temporally, nasally).

Abnormal Findings:

Hesitancy, squinting, leaning forward, misreading letters.

The larger the denominator, the poorer the vision. If vision is poorer than 20/30, refer to an eye specialist. Impaired vision occurs with refractive error, opacity in the media (cornea, lens, vitreous), or disorder in the retina or optic pathway.

Presbyopia, the decrease in power of accommodation with aging, is suggested when the person moves the card farther away.

Normal Range of Findings	Abnormal Findings

Ask the person to say "now" as the wiggling fingertip is first seen; this should be just as you also see it.

If the person is unable to see as you do, the test suggests peripheral field loss. Refer to an eye specialist for more precise testing.

Inspect Extraocular Muscle Function

Diagnostic Positions Test

Leading the eyes through the 6 *cardinal positions of gaze* elicits any muscle weakness during movement. Ask the person to hold the head steady and follow the movement of your finger, only with the eyes. Hold your finger back about 12 inches so the person can focus on it comfortably; move it to each of the 6 positions, hold it momentarily, then move it back to center. Progress clockwise (Fig. 7.4). A normal response is parallel tracking of the object with both eyes.

Eye movement is not parallel. Failure to follow in a certain direction indicates weakness of an extraocular muscle (EOM) or dysfunction of the cranial nerve that innervates it.

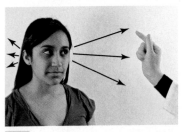

7.4

In addition to parallel movement, note any **nystagmus,** a fine oscillating movement best seen around the iris. Mild nystagmus at extreme lateral gaze is normal; nystagmus at any other position is not.

Finally note that the upper eyelid continues to overlap the superior part of the iris, even during downward movement.

Nystagmus occurs with disease of the semicircular canals in the ears, a paretic eye muscle, multiple sclerosis, or brain lesion.

A white rim of sclera between the lid and the iris, referred to as "lid lag," occurs with hyperthyroidism.

Normal Range of Findings	Abnormal Findings

Inspect External Ocular Structures

General

Note the person's ability to move around the room with vision functioning well enough to avoid obstacles and respond to your directions. The facial expression is relaxed with adequate vision.

Groping with hands.

Squinting or craning forward.

Eyebrows

Normally the eyebrows are present bilaterally, move symmetrically as the facial expression changes, and have no scaling or lesions.

Unequal or absent movement with nerve damage.

Scaling with seborrhea.

Eyelids and Lashes

The upper lids normally overlap the superior part of the iris and approximate completely when closed. The skin is intact without redness, swelling, discharge, or lesions.

The palpebral fissures are horizontal in non-Asians, whereas palpebral fissures of Asians normally have an upward slant.

The eyelashes are evenly distributed along the lid margins and curve outward.

Lid lag occurs with hyperthyroidism. Incomplete closure creates risk for corneal damage.
Ptosis—drooping of upper lid as with myasthenia gravis.

Periorbital edema, lesions.

Ectropion and entropion (Table 7.2, p. 78).

Eyeballs

The eyeballs are aligned normally with no protrusion or sunken appearance. Blacks may normally have a slight protrusion of the eyeball beyond the supraorbital ridge.

Exophthalmos—protruding eyes (see Table 7.2).
Enophthalmos—sunken eyes.

Conjunctiva and Sclera

Ask the person to look up. Using your thumbs, slide the lower lids down along the bony orbital rim. Take care not to push against the eyeball (Fig. 7.5). Inspect the exposed area. The eyeball looks moist and glossy. Numerous small blood vessels normally show through the transparent conjunctiva. Otherwise the conjunctivae are clear and show the normal color of the

Normal Range of Findings	Abnormal Findings

structure below—pink over the lower lids and white over the sclera. Note any color change, swelling, or lesions.

General reddening (see Table 7.2).
Cyanosis of the lower lids.
Pallor near the outer canthus of the lower lid may indicate anemia (the inner canthus normally contains less pigment).

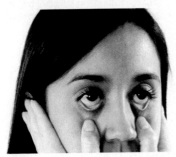

7.5

The sclera is china white, although occasionally it is gray-blue or "muddy" color in blacks. Dark-skinned people may have small brown macules (like freckles) on the sclera; do not confuse these with foreign bodies or petechiae. Blacks may have yellowish fatty deposits beneath the lids away from the cornea. Do not confuse these yellow spots with the overall scleral yellowing that accompanies jaundice.

Scleral icterus is a yellowing of the sclera extending up to the cornea, indicating jaundice.
Tenderness, foreign body, discharge, or lesions.

Inspect Anterior Eyeball Structures

Cornea and Lens

Shine a light from the side across the cornea and check for smoothness and clarity. There should be no opacities (cloudiness) in the cornea, the anterior chamber, or in the lens behind the pupil. Do not confuse **arcus senilis** with an opacity. This is a normal finding in older adults and is described on p. 74.

A corneal abrasion causes irregular ridges in reflected light, usually visible only with fluorescein stain.

Iris and Pupils

The iris normally has a round, regular shape and an even coloration.

Normal Range of Findings	Abnormal Findings

Normally the pupils appear round, regular, and of equal size. In adults resting size is from 3 to 5 mm. A small number of people (5%) have pupils of two different sizes, a condition called **anisocoria.**

Irregular shape.

Pupils with unequal size occur with a central nervous system injury.

To test the **pupillary light reflex,** darken the room and ask the person to gaze into the distance. (This dilates the pupils.) Advance a light in from the side,[a] and note the response. Normally you will see (1) constriction of the pupil on the same side (a *direct light reflex*), and (2) simultaneous constriction of the other pupil (a *consensual light reflex*).

Dilated pupils.
Dilated and fixed pupils.
Constricted pupils.
Unequal or no response to light (Table 7.3).

Test for **accommodation** by asking the person to focus on a distant object. This process dilates the pupils. Then have the person shift the gaze to a near object such as your finger held about 7 to 8 cm (3 inches) from the nose.

A normal response includes (1) pupillary constriction and (2) convergence of the axes of the eyes.

Absence of constriction or convergence.
Asymmetric response.

Record the normal response to these maneuvers as PERRLA, or *Pupils Equal, Round, React to Light,* and *Accommodation.*

ADVANCED PRACTICE TECHNIQUES

Inspect the Ocular Fundus

Darken the room to help dilate the pupils. Remove eyeglasses from yourself or the other person; they obstruct close movement, and you can compensate for their correction by using the diopter setting. Contact lenses can be left in.

---

[a]Always advance the light in from the *side* to test the light reflex. If you advance from the front, the pupils will constrict to accommodate for near vision. Thus you do not know what the pure response to the light would have been.

Normal Range of Findings	Abnormal Findings

Select the large round aperture with the white light of the ophthalmoscope for routine examination. If the pupils are small, use the smaller white light.

Tell the person, "Please keep looking at that light switch [or mark] on the wall across the room, even though my head will get in the way." Staring at a distant fixed object helps dilate the pupils and hold the retinal structures still.

Match sides with the person: that is, hold the ophthalmoscope in your *right* hand up to your *right* eye to view the person's *right* eye (Fig. 7.6). You must do this to avoid bumping noses during the procedure. Place your free hand on the person's shoulder or forehead.

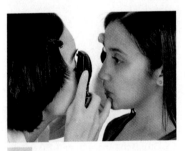

7.6

Systematically inspect the structures in the ocular fundus: (1) optic disc, (2) retinal vessels, (3) general background, and (4) macula (see Fig. 7.3). (Note that the illustration shows a large area of the fundus. Your actual view through the ophthalmoscope is much smaller, slightly larger than 1 disc diameter.)

Optic Disc

The most prominent landmark is the optic disc, located on the nasal side of the retina. Explore these characteristics:

Normal Range of Findings	Abnormal Findings
1. Color—Creamy yellow-orange to pink	Pallor. Hyperemia.
2. Shape—Round or oval	Irregular.
3. Margins—Distinct, sharply demarcated, although the nasal edge may be slightly fuzzy	Blurred margins.
4. Cup-to-disc ratio—Distinctness varies. When visible, cup is a brighter yellow-white than the rest of the disc. Its width is not more than one-half of the disc diameter (DD).	Cup extending to the disc border (see Table 15.9, p. 314, in Jarvis: *Physical Examination and Health Assessment,* 8th ed.).

Retinal Vessels

Follow a paired artery and vein out to the periphery in the four quadrants (see Fig. 7.3), noting these points:

1. Number—A paired artery and vein pass to each quadrant. Vessels look straighter at the nasal side.	Absence of major vessels.
2. Color—Arteries are brighter red than veins. They also have the arterial light reflex, a thin stripe of light down the middle.	
3. A:V ratio—The ratio comparing the artery-to-vein width is 2:3 or 4:5.	Arteries too constricted. Veins dilated.
4. Caliber—Arteries and veins show a regular decrease in caliber as they extend to periphery.	Focal constriction. Neovascularization.
5. Arteriovenous (AV) crossing—An artery and vein may cross paths. This is not significant if within 2 DD of disc and if no sign of interruption in blood flow. There should be no indenting or displacing of vessel.	Crossings more than 2 DD away from disc. Nicking or pinching of underlying vessel. Vessel engorged peripheral to crossing.
6. Tortuosity—Mild vessel twisting when present in both eyes is usually congenital and not significant.	Extreme tortuosity or marked asymmetry in two eyes.
7. Pulsations—Present in veins near the disc as their drainage meets the intermittent pressure of arterial systole (often hard to see).	Absent pulsations (see Table 15.9, p. 314, in Jarvis: *Physical Examination and Health Assessment,* 8th ed.).

General Background of the Fundus

The color normally varies from light red to dark brown–red, generally corresponding with the person's skin color.

Normal Range of Findings	Abnormal Findings

There should be no lesions obstructing the retinal structures.

Abnormal lesions—hemorrhages, exudates, microaneurysms.

Macula

The macula is 1 DD in size and is located 2 DD temporal to the disc. Inspect this area last in the funduscopic examination. A bright light on this area of central vision causes some watering, discomfort, and pupillary constriction. Note that the normal color of the area is somewhat darker than the rest of the fundus but even and homogeneous. Clumped pigment may occur with aging.

Clumped pigment occurs with trauma or retinal detachment.

Hemorrhage or exudate in the macula occurs with macular degeneration.

❖ DEVELOPMENTAL COMPETENCE

Infants and Children. Test a newborn's **light perception** using the blink reflex; neonates blink in response to bright light. The pupillary light reflex also shows that the pupils constrict in response to light.

Testing for **strabismus** (squint, crossed eye) is an important screening measure during early childhood. Untreated strabismus can lead to permanent visual damage, called *amblyopia ex anopsia*. Early recognition and treatment are essential.

Check the **corneal light reflex** by shining a light toward the child's eyes. The light should be reflected at exactly the same spot in the two corneas. Some asymmetry (where one light falls off center) under age 6 months is normal.

Many infants have an **epicanthal fold,** an excess skinfold extending over the inner corner of the eye, partly or totally overlapping the inner canthus. This occurs frequently in Asian children and in 20% of whites. Epicanthal folds give a false appearance of malalignment, called *pseudostrabismus,* but the corneal light reflex is normal.

Absent blinking.

Absent pupillary light reflex, especially after 3 weeks, indicates blindness.

Diagnosis after age 6 years has a poor prognosis.

Asymmetry in the corneal light reflex after 6 months is abnormal, and the infant must be referred.

Normal Range of Findings	Abnormal Findings
Asian infants normally have an upward slant of the palpebral fissures. Entropion, a turning inward of the eyelid, is normally found in some Asian children. If the lashes do not abrade the cornea, it is not significant.	An upward lateral slope together with epicanthal folds and hypertelorism (large spacing between the eyes) occurs with Down syndrome.

The Aging Adult

The eyebrows may show a loss of the outer one-third of hair. The remaining brow hair is coarse. Because of atrophy of elastic tissue, the skin around the eyes may show wrinkles or crow's feet. The upper lid may be so elongated as to rest on the lashes (Table 7.1 on p. 75).

The eyes may appear sunken because of atrophy of the orbital fat. The orbital fat may also herniate, causing bulging at the lower lids and inner third of the upper lids.

Atrophy of the levator palpebrae muscle causes a partial ptosis. In contrast with the baggy lids previously described, ptosis is an actual drooping.

The lower lid may drop away (i.e., **ectropion**). Then tears cannot drain into the out-turned puncta. Alternately, **entropion,** or a turning inward, may irritate the eye from friction of lashes (see Table 7.2 on p. 78).

Tear production may decrease, causing the eyes to look dry and lusterless and the person to report a burning sensation. **Pingueculae** commonly show on the sclera (see Table 7.1). These yellowish elevated nodules are caused by a thickening of the bulbar conjunctiva from prolonged exposure to sun, wind, and dust. Pingueculae appear at the 3 o'clock and 9 o'clock positions, first on the nasal side and then on the temporal side.

Distinguish pingueculae from the abnormal **pterygium,** an opacity also on the bulbar conjunctiva, but which grows over the cornea and may block vision.

The cornea may look cloudy with age. **Arcus senilis** is commonly seen around the cornea (see Table 7.1). This is a gray-white arc or circle around the limbus caused by deposition of lipid material. As more lipid accumulates, the cornea may look thickened and raised, but the arcus has no effect on vision.

Normal Range of Findings	Abnormal Findings

Xanthelasma are soft, raised yellow plaques occurring on the lids of the inner canthus (see Table 7.1). These commonly occur around age 50 and older, more frequently in women. Xanthelasma occur with both high and normal blood levels of cholesterol and have no pathologic significance.

Pupils are small, and the pupillary light reflex may be slowed. The lens loses transparency and appears opaque.

TABLE 7.1   Aging Eye Changes

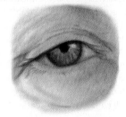

Relaxation of skin of upper eyelid

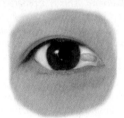

Pinguecula

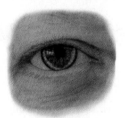

Arcus senilis

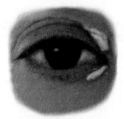

Xanthelasma

© Pat Thomas, 2010.

In the ocular fundus the blood vessels appear pale, narrow, and attenuated. Arterioles appear pale and straight, with a narrow light reflex. More AV crossing defects occur.

Normal Range of Findings	Abnormal Findings
A normal development on the retinal surface is **drusen,** or benign degenerative hyaline deposits. They are small, round yellow dots that are scattered haphazardly on the retina. Although they do not occur in a pattern, drusen are usually symmetrically placed in the two eyes. They have no effect on vision.	Drusen are easily confused with the abnormal finding of *hard exudates* (see Table 15.10, p. 315, in Jarvis: *Physical Examination and Health Assessment,* 8th ed.).

HEALTH PROMOTION AND PATIENT TEACHING

(To all adults over 40 years) *I want to refer you to an eye specialist for screening for glaucoma. This is a progressive eye disease that affects over 2 million Americans and robs them of peripheral (side) vision. Most people with glaucoma have no symptoms and do not know they have the disease, but it can be treated. An eye specialist can screen you with specific equipment that we do not have in the hospital or in the primary care office.*

Glaucoma is a set of progressive eye neuropathies that can lead to severe visual field loss and blindness. It is the leading cause of irreversible blindness among blacks and Hispanics (Gupta & Chen, 2016). Glaucoma can reduce peripheral vision without yet harming central vision. Those who have glaucoma who are not blind still may have limited function, e.g., decreased ability to drive a car or to read.

Summary Checklist: Eyes

1. **Test visual acuity:**
   Snellen eye chart
   Near vision (those ≥40 years or those having difficulty reading)
2. **Test visual fields:**
   Confrontation test
3. **Inspect EOM function:**
   Corneal light reflex
   Diagnostic positions test
4. **Inspect external eye structures:**
   General
   Eyebrows
   Eyelids and lashes
   Eyeball alignment
   Conjunctivae and sclerae

5. **Inspect anterior eyeball structures:**
   Cornea and lens
   Iris and pupil
   Size, shape, and equality
   Pupillary light reflex
   Accommodation
6. **Inspect the ocular fundus:**
   Optic disc (color, shape, margins, cup : disc ratio)
   Retinal vessels (number, color, artery : vein [A : V] ratio, caliber, AV crossings, tortuosity, pulsations)
   General background (color, integrity)
   Macula

DOCUMENTATION

Sample Charting

SUBJECTIVE

Vision reported "good" with no recent change. No eye pain, no inflammation, no discharge, no lesions. Wears no corrective lenses, vision last tested 1 year PTA; test for glaucoma at that time was normal.

OBJECTIVE

Snellen chart—Right 20/20, Left 20/20 −1. Fields normal by confrontation. Corneal light reflex symmetric bilaterally. Diagnostic positions test shows EOMs intact. Brows and lashes present. No ptosis. Conjunctiva clear. Sclera white. No lesions. PERRLA.

Fundi—Red reflex present bilaterally. Discs flat with sharp margins. Vessels present in all quadrants without crossing defects. Retinal background has even color with no hemorrhages or exudates. Macula has even color.

ASSESSMENT

Healthy vision function
Healthy eye structures

ABNORMAL FINDINGS

TABLE 7.2	Abnormalities in the Eyelids

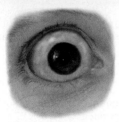

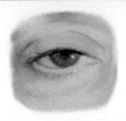

Exophthalmos (Protruding Eyes)
Exophthalmos is a forward displacement associated with thyroid disease. Note "lid lag," i.e., the upper lid rests well above the limbus, and white sclera is visible.

Ptosis (Drooping Upper Lid)
Ptosis occurs from neuromuscular weakness (e.g., myasthenia gravis), oculomotor cranial nerve III damage, or sympathetic nerve damage (e.g., Horner syndrome).

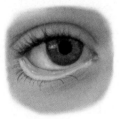

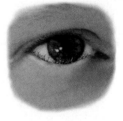

Ectropion
The lower lid is loose and rolling out and does not approximate to the eyeball. Puncta cannot siphon tears effectively; therefore excess tearing results. Exposed palpebral conjunctiva increases risk for inflammation.

Entropion
The lower lid rolls in as a result of spasm of lids or contraction of scar tissue. Lashes may irritate cornea. Symptoms are foreign body sensation, tearing, and red eye.

Continued

TABLE 7.2 Abnormalities in the Eyelids—cont'd

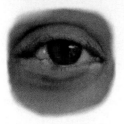

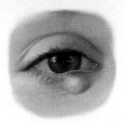

Hordeolum (Stye)

Hordeolum is a localized staphylococcal infection of the hair follicles at the lid margin. It is painful, red, and swollen and resembles a pustule at the lid margin.

Chalazion

A beady nodule protruding on the lid, chalazion is an infection or retention cyst of a meibomian gland. It is a nontender, firm, discrete swelling with freely movable skin overlying the nodule. If it becomes inflamed, it points inside and not on the lid margin (in contrast with a stye).

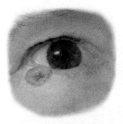

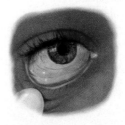

Basal Cell Carcinoma

Carcinoma is rare, but it occurs most often on the lower lid. It looks like a papule with an ulcerated center. The edges are rolled out and pearly.

Conjunctivitis

Infection of the conjunctiva shows red, beefy-looking vessels at the periphery but looks clearer around the iris. This is common from bacterial or viral infection, allergy, or chemical irritant. It often accompanies an upper respiratory infection. Purulent discharge accompanies bacterial infection.

Images © Pat Thomas, 2010.

TABLE 7.3	Abnormalities in the Pupil

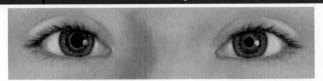

Unequal Pupil Size—Anisocoria

Although anisocoria exists normally in 5% of the population, a person with this condition may have central nervous system disease.

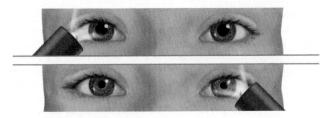

Monocular Blindness

When light is directed to the blind eye, there is no response. When light is directed to the normal eye, both pupils constrict (direct and consensual response to light) as long as the oculomotor nerve is intact.

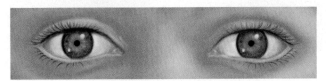

Constricted and Fixed Pupils—Miosis

Miosis occurs with the use of pilocarpine drops for glaucoma treatment, with the use of narcotics, with iritis, and with brain damage of the pons.

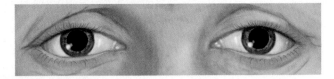

Dilated and Fixed Pupils—Mydriasis

Enlarged pupils occur with stimulation of the sympathetic nervous system, as a reaction of sympathomimetic drugs, with use of dilating drops, with acute glaucoma, and with past or recent trauma. Enlarged pupils may also indicate central nervous system injury, cardiac arrest, or deep anesthesia.

CHAPTER 8

Ears

ANATOMY

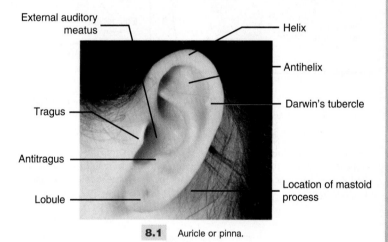

External auditory meatus

Helix

Antihelix

Darwin's tubercle

Tragus

Antitragus

Lobule

Location of mastoid process

8.1 Auricle or pinna.

The ear is the sensory organ for hearing and maintaining equilibrium. The external ear is the **auricle,** or **pinna**, and consists of movable cartilage and skin (Fig. 8.1).

The external ear funnels sound into its opening, the **external auditory canal.** The canal is a cul-de-sac, 2.5 to 3 cm long in the adult, and has a slight S-curve (Fig. 8.2).

The middle ear is a tiny, air-filled cavity inside the temporal bone containing the tiny auditory ossicles: the *malleus, incus,* and *stapes.*

The inner ear contains the *bony labyrinth,* which holds the sensory organs for equilibrium and hearing.

The **tympanic membrane,** or **eardrum,** separates the external and middle ear (Fig. 8.3). It is translucent,

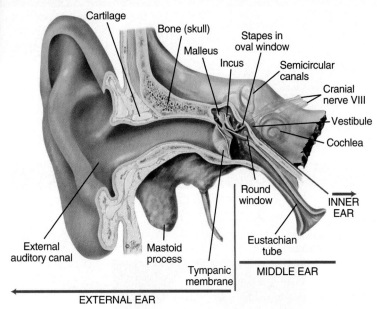

8.2   Internal ear structures.   (© Pat Thomas, 2010.)

with a pearly gray color and a prominent cone of light in the anteroinferior quadrant, which is the reflection of the otoscope light.

The parts of the malleus show through the translucent drum; these are the *umbo,* the *manubrium,* and the *short process.*

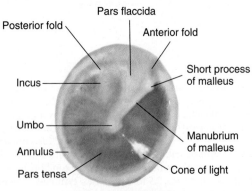

TYMPANIC MEMBRANE

8.3

CULTURE AND GENETICS

Cerumen is determined genetically and comes in two major types: (1) dry cerumen, which is gray and flaky and frequently forms a thin mass in the ear canal; and (2) wet cerumen, which is honey-to–dark brown and moist. The wet cerumen phenotype occurs more often in Caucasians and African Americans, whereas the dry cerumen is more frequent in East Asians and American Indians (Prokop-Prigge et al., 2014).

Middle ear infection (otitis media, or OM) occurs because of obstruction of the eustachian tube or passage of nasopharyngeal secretions (containing virus or bacteria) into the middle ear. Acute OM is so common that up to 60% of children have an episode during the first year of life, and by age 3 years up to 83% have had an episode (Rosa-Olivares et al., 2015). However, ambulatory visits for acute OM have decreased, probably because of an increase in smoke-free households and vehicles. Also, hospital admissions for acute OM have decreased since the addition of pneumococcal vaccination to the early childhood schedule, as well as the influenza vaccination (Tawfik et al., 2017).

SUBJECTIVE DATA

1. Earaches
2. Infections
3. Discharge
4. Hearing loss
5. Environmental noise
6. Tinnitus
7. Vertigo
8. Patient-centered care (hearing last checked, method of cleaning ears)

OBJECTIVE DATA

PREPARATION
Position the adult sitting up straight with his or her head at your eye level.

EQUIPMENT NEEDED
Otoscope with bright light (fresh batteries give off white, not yellow, light)
Pneumatic bulb attachment, sometimes used with infants or young children

Normal Range of Findings	Abnormal Findings
Inspect and Palpate the External Ear	
Size and Shape	
The ears are of equal size bilaterally with no swelling or thickening.	*Microtia*—Ears smaller than 4 cm vertically. *Macrotia*—Ears larger than 10 cm. Edema.

Normal Range of Findings	Abnormal Findings

Skin Condition

The skin is intact, with no lumps or lesions. *Darwin tubercle,* a small painless nodule at the helix, is sometimes present. This is a congenital variation and is not significant (see Fig. 8.1).

Reddened, excessively warm skin indicates inflammation.

Crusts and scaling occur with otitis externa and with eczema, contact dermatitis, and seborrhea.

Enlarged tender lymph nodes in the region indicate inflammation of the pinna or mastoid process.

Tophi, sebaceous crust, chondrodermatitis, keloid, carcinoma (see Table 16.2, p. 335, in Jarvis: *Physical Examination and Health Assessment,* 8th ed.).

Tenderness

The pinna and tragus should feel firm, and movement should produce no pain. Palpating the mastoid process should be painless.

Pain with movement occurs with otitis externa and furuncle.

Pain at the mastoid process may indicate mastoiditis or lymphadenitis of the posterior auricular node.

External Auditory Meatus

There should be no swelling, redness, or discharge.

A sticky yellow discharge accompanies otitis externa, or it may indicate otitis media if the drum has ruptured.

Some cerumen is usually present. The color varies from gray-yellow to light brown and black, and the texture varies from moist and waxy to dry and desiccated.

Impacted cerumen is a common cause of conductive hearing loss.

The Otoscopic Examination

Choose the largest speculum that fits comfortably. Tilt the person's head slightly away from you toward the opposite shoulder. This method brings the obliquely sloping eardrum into better view.

Pull the pinna up and back on an adult or older child (Fig. 8.4); this helps straighten the S-shape of the canal. (Pull the pinna down on an infant or child younger than 3 years of age.)

Normal Range of Findings	Abnormal Findings

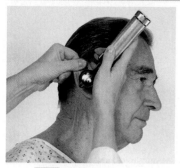

8.4   Using an otoscope.

Hold the otoscope upside down along your fingers and have the dorsum (back) of your hand along the person's cheek, braced to steady the otoscope (see Fig. 8.4).

External Canal

Note any redness and swelling, lesions, foreign bodies, or discharge. If any discharge is present, note the color and odor. (Also clean any discharge off the speculum before examining the other ear to avoid contamination with possibly infectious material.) For a person with a hearing aid, note any irritation on the canal wall from poorly fitting ear molds.

Redness and swelling occur with otitis externa; the canal may be completely closed with swelling.

Purulent otorrhea suggests otitis externa or otitis media if the drum has ruptured.

Frank blood or clear watery drainage (cerebrospinal fluid leak) after trauma suggests basal skull fracture and warrants immediate referral. Cerebrospinal fluid feels oily and tests positive for glucose.

Foreign body, exostosis, polyp, furuncle (see Table 16.4, p. 338, in Jarvis: *Physical Examination and Health Assessment,* 8th ed.).

Normal Range of Findings	Abnormal Findings

Tympanic Membrane

Color and Characteristics. The normal eardrum is shiny and translucent, with a pearl-gray color (see Fig. 8.3). The cone-shaped light reflex is prominent in the anterior inferior quadrant (at the 5-o'clock position in the right drum and at the 7-o'clock position in the left drum). This is the reflection of the otoscope light. Sections of the malleus are visible through the translucent drum—the umbo, manubrium, and short process. (Infrequently the incus behind the drum shows as a whitish haze in the upper posterior area.) At the periphery the annulus looks whiter and denser.

Yellow-amber color of the drum occurs with serous otitis media.
Red color occurs with acute otitis media.

Absent or distorted landmarks.
Air/fluid level or air bubbles behind the drum indicate serous otitis media (Table 8.1, p. 91).

Position. The eardrum is flat and slightly pulled in at the center.

Retracted drum due to vacuum in middle ear.
Bulging drum from otitis media.

Integrity of Membrane. The normal tympanic membrane is intact. Some adults may show scarring or a dense white patch on the drum as a sequela of repeated ear infections.

Perforation shows as a dark oval area or as a larger opening on the drum (see Table 8.1).

Vesicles on drum.

Test Hearing Acuity

Whispered Voice Test

Stand behind the person at arm's length (2 feet). Test one ear at a time while masking hearing in the other ear by placing one finger on the tragus and pushing it in and out of the auditory meatus. Exhale fully and whisper slowly a set of 3 random numbers and letters such as "5, B, 6." Normally the person repeats each number/letter correctly after you say it. If the response is not correct, repeat the whispered test using a different combination of 3 numbers and letters. A passing score is correctly repeating at least 4 out of a possible 6 numbers/letters. Assess the other ear using another set of whispered items, "4, K, 2."

The person is unable to hear whispered sounds. A whisper is a high-frequency sound and is used to detect high-tone loss.

Normal Range of Findings	Abnormal Findings

Tuning Fork Tests

Tuning fork tests measure hearing by air conduction (AC) or bone conduction (BC) in which the sound vibrates through the cranial bones to the inner ear. The AC route through the ear canal and middle ear is usually more sensitive. Traditionally these tests were taught; yet evidence shows that both the Weber and Rinne tuning fork tests do not yield precise or reliable data. Close to 40% of normal hearing people lateralize the Weber test. Thus these tests should not be used for general screening.

With documented hearing loss, these tests may help distinguish conductive loss from sensorineural loss (see Table 16.7, Tuning Fork Tests, p. 342, in Jarvis: *Physical Examination and Health Assessment*, 8th ed.), but they cannot distinguish normal hearing from a sensorineural loss in both ears (McGee, 2018).

DEVELOPMENTAL COMPETENCE

Infants and Young Children

The top of the pinna should match an imaginary line extending from the corner of the eye to the occiput, and the ear should be positioned within 10 degrees of vertical.

Low-set ears are found with trisomy 13, 18, 21. Large, prominent ears; misshapen ears; and creases on earlobes are nonspecific. Preauricular skin tags may occur alone or with other facial anomalies.

Remember to pull the pinna straight down on an infant or child younger than 3 years old. This method matches the slope of the ear canal.

When examining an infant or a young child, a pneumatic bulb attachment enables you to direct a light puff of air toward the drum to assess vibratility (Fig. 8.5). For a secure seal choose the largest speculum that fits the ear canal without causing pain. A rubber tip on the end of the speculum gives a better seal. Give a small pump to the bulb (positive pressure) and release it (negative pressure). Normally the tympanic membrane moves inward with a slight puff and outward with a slight release.

An abnormal response is no movement of the eardrum. Drum hypomobility indicates effusion or a high vacuum in the middle ear. For the newborn's first 6 weeks, drum immobility is the best indicator of middle ear infection.

Normal Range of Findings	Abnormal Findings

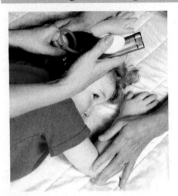

8.5 Using an otoscope with pneumatic bulb attachment.

Normally the tympanic membrane is intact. In a child being treated for chronic otitis media, you may note the presence of a tympanostomy tube in the central part of the drum. It is inserted surgically to equalize pressure and drain secretions. Note a foreign body in a child's ear canal such as a small stone or bead.

Foreign body (see Table 16.4, p. 338, in Jarvis: *Physical Examination and Health Assessment,* 8th ed.).

The Aging Adult

Earlobes may be pendulous with linear wrinkling. Coarse, wiry hairs may be present at the opening of the ear canal. During otoscopy the drum may be whiter in color and more opaque—duller than in the younger adult. It also may look thickened.

High-tone frequency hearing loss is apparent for those affected with **presbycusis,** the hearing loss that occurs with aging. This condition is revealed by difficulty hearing whispered sounds in the voice test and difficulty hearing consonants during conversational speech.

Normal Range of Findings	Abnormal Findings
For more information on ear and hearing assessment, see Chapter 16 in Jarvis: *Physical Examination and Health Assessment,* 8th ed., pp. 317-344.	

HEALTH PROMOTION AND PATIENT TEACHING

"Your newborn baby's hearing will be checked before the baby leaves the hospital or during the first month of life. This is important because the crucial time to learn language is in the first 3 years of life as the brain develops and matures. Hearing loss is not common, but if there is a loss, research shows that children who get help early develop better language skills than those who do not get help." The 1-3-6 program of universal newborn hearing screening (NIH, 2017) consists of the following:

1 = All newborns are screened for hearing loss before they leave the hospital or within 1 month of life.

3 = All infants who do not pass the hearing screening should be scheduled immediately for a follow-up appointment with a pediatric audiologist. This examination must happen by age 3 months.

6 = If the follow-up examination confirms that the baby has hearing loss, the baby must receive appropriate interventions by 6 months of age, including hearing devices and early communication intervention (e.g., lipreading, signed English, American Sign Language, or others).

Summary Checklist: Ears

1. **Inspect external ear:**
   Size and shape of auricle
   Position and alignment on head
   Skin condition
       Color, lumps, lesions
       Movement of auricle and
          tragus (for tenderness)
       External auditory meatus
       Size, swelling, redness,
          discharge, cerumen,
          lesions, foreign bodies
2. **Otoscopic examination:**
   External canal
       Cerumen, discharge, foreign
          bodies, lesions

   Redness or swelling of canal
       wall
   Tympanic membrane
       Color and characteristics
       Note position (flat, bulging,
          retracted)
       Integrity of membrane (no
          perforations)
3. **Test hearing acuity:**
   Note behavioral response to
       conversational speech
   Whispered voice test

DOCUMENTATION

Sample Charting

SUBJECTIVE

States hearing is good, no earaches, infections, discharge, hearing loss, tinnitus, or vertigo.

OBJECTIVE

Pinna: Skin intact with no masses, lesions, tenderness, or discharge.

Otoscope: External canals are clear with no redness, swelling, lesions, foreign body, or discharge. Both TMs are pearly gray in color, with light reflex and landmarks intact, no perforations.

Hearing: Responds appropriately to conversation. Whispered sounds heard bilaterally.

ASSESSMENT

Healthy ear structures
Hearing accurate

ABNORMAL FINDINGS

TABLE 8.1	Ear Canal or Tympanic Membrane Abnormalities

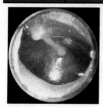

Retracted Drum

Landmarks look more prominent. Malleus handle looks shorter and more horizontal. Short process is very prominent. Light reflex is absent or distorted. Drum is dull and lusterless and does not move. Signs indicate obstructed eustachian tube and serous otitis media.

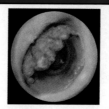

Excessive Cerumen

Excessive cerumen is impacted because of a narrow tortuous canal or faulty cleaning method. It may appear as a round ball partially or totally obscuring the drum. Total occlusion results in ear fullness and impaired hearing.

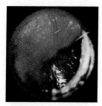

Acute Otitis Media

An absent or distorted light reflex is an early sign. Redness and bulging are first noted in superior drum (pars flaccida), along with earache and fever. Then fiery red bulging of entire drum occurs, with deep throbbing pain, fever, and transient hearing loss. Pneumatic otoscopy reveals drum hypomobility.

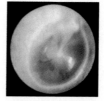

Otitis Media with Effusion

An amber-yellow drum, an air/fluid level with fine black dividing line, or air bubbles visible behind drum. Symptoms are feeling of fullness, transient hearing loss, popping sound with swallowing. Also called *serous otitis media* and *glue ear*.

Continued

TABLE 8.1	Ear Canal or Tympanic Membrane Abnormalities—cont'd

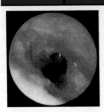 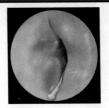

Perforation

Drum rupture from increased pressure or trauma. Usually perforation appears as round or oval darkened area on drum, but in this photo perforation is very large. Central perforations occur in pars tensa, marginal perforations at the annulus.

Otitis Externa

Severe swelling of canal; inflammation; tenderness. An infection of the outer ear, with severe painful movement of pinna and tragus, redness and swelling of pinna and canal, scanty purulent discharge, scaling, itching, fever, and enlarged tender regional lymph nodes. Hearing is normal or slightly diminished.

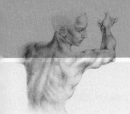

CHAPTER 9

Nose, Mouth, and Throat

ANATOMY

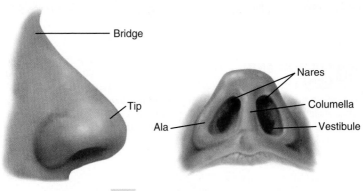

9.1 External nose structures. (© Pat Thomas, 2006.)

The **nose** is the first segment of the respiratory system. It warms, moistens, and filters the inhaled air; and it is the sensory organ for smell.

The oval openings at the base of the nose are the *nares* (Fig. 9.1). The *columella* divides the two nares and is continuous inside with the nasal septum.

Inside, the **nasal cavity** is large and extends back over the roof of the mouth (Fig. 9.2). Nasal mucosa appears redder than oral mucosa because of the rich blood supply present to warm the inhaled air.

The lateral walls of each nasal cavity contain three bony projections—the *turbinates*. They increase the surface area so more blood vessels are available to warm, humidify, and filter the inhaled air.

The **mouth** is the first segment of the digestive system and an airway for the respiratory system (Fig. 9.3). It contains the teeth and gums, tongue, and three pairs of salivary glands. The hard (bony) palate is whitish; the more posterior soft palate is an arch of muscle that is pinker and mobile.

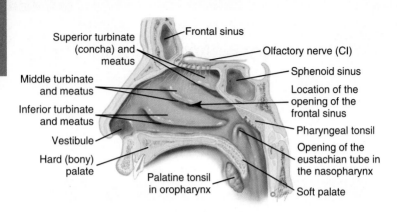

Superior turbinate (concha) and meatus

Middle turbinate and meatus

Inferior turbinate and meatus

Vestibule

Hard (bony) palate

Palatine tonsil in oropharynx

Frontal sinus

Olfactory nerve (CI)

Sphenoid sinus

Location of the opening of the frontal sinus

Pharyngeal tonsil

Opening of the eustachian tube in the nasopharynx

Soft palate

RIGHT LATERAL WALL—NASAL CAVITY

9.2 Internal nose structures. (© Pat Thomas, 2006.)

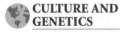

CULTURE AND GENETICS

The incidence of **cleft lip** with or without **cleft palate** is one in every 940 births in the United States; isolated cleft palate is less common (ASHA, 2017). Rates are higher in Asians and American Indians (1:500 births) and lower in African heritage births (1:2500). **Dental caries** (tooth decay) is an infectious process that occurs when bacteria interact with carbohydrates in sweet drinks and food. There has been

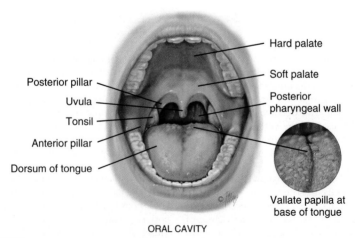

Posterior pillar

Uvula

Tonsil

Anterior pillar

Dorsum of tongue

Hard palate

Soft palate

Posterior pharyngeal wall

Vallate papilla at base of tongue

ORAL CAVITY

9.3 Mouth structures. (© Pat Thomas, 2010.)

a significant increase in decay in the United States: 42% of children ages 2 to 11 years have dental caries in their primary teeth; 23% of children ages 2 to 11 years have untreated dental caries; and 21% of children ages 6 to 11 years have dental caries in their permanent teeth (NIH, 2014). In all groups, black and Hispanic children and children in lower-income families have more decay.

SUBJECTIVE DATA

Nose
1. Discharge
2. Frequent colds (upper respiratory infections, or URI)
3. Sinus pain
4. Trauma
5. Epistaxis (nosebleeds)
6. Allergies
7. Altered smell

Mouth and Throat
8. Sores or lesions
9. Sore throat
10. Bleeding gums
11. Toothache
12. Hoarseness
13. Dysphagia
14. Altered taste
15. Smoking, alcohol consumption
16. Patient-centered care (dental care pattern, dentures or appliances)

OBJECTIVE DATA

PREPARATION

Position the person sitting up straight with his or her head at your eye level. Remove any dentures.

EQUIPMENT NEEDED

Otoscope with short, wide-tipped nasal speculum attachment or nasal speculum and penlight
Tongue blade
Cotton gauze pad (4 × 4 inches)
Gloves

Normal Range of Findings	Abnormal Findings
Inspect and Palpate the Nose The nose is symmetric, in the midline, and in proportion to other facial features. Inspect for any deformity, asymmetry, inflammation, or skin lesions. Test the patency of the nostrils. This reveals any obstruction, which can be explored later with the nasal speculum.	Absence of sniff indicates obstruction, e.g., nasal polyps, rhinitis.

Normal Range of Findings	Abnormal Findings

Nasal Cavity

Attach the short, wide-tipped speculum to the otoscope head and insert into the nasal vestibule, avoiding pressure on the nasal septum (Fig. 9.4).

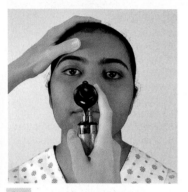

9.4 Viewing naris through nasal speculum.

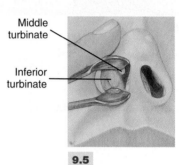

Middle turbinate

Inferior turbinate

9.5

Inspect the nasal mucosa, noting its normal red color and smooth moist surface (Fig. 9.5). Note any swelling, discharge, bleeding, or foreign body (Table 9.1, p. 103).

Rhinitis—Nasal mucosa is swollen and bright red with a URI.

Discharge is common with rhinitis and sinusitis, varying from watery and copious to thick, purulent, and green-yellow.

With chronic allergy, mucosa looks swollen, boggy, pale, and gray.

For more information on abnormalities of the nose, see Table 17.1, p. 367, in Jarvis: *Physical Examination and Health Assessment,* 8th ed.

Observe the nasal septum for deviation, perforation, or bleeding. A deviated septum is common and not significant unless airflow is obstructed.

A deviated septum looks like a hump or shelf in one nasal cavity.

Perforation is seen as a spot of light from penlight shining in other naris.

Epistaxis commonly comes from the anterior septum.

Inspect the turbinates, the bony ridges curving down from the lateral walls. The middle and inferior turbinates appear the same light red color as the nasal mucosa. Note any swelling

Normal Range of Findings	Abnormal Findings

but do not try to push the speculum past it. Turbinates are quite vascular and tender if touched.

Note any polyps, and distinguish them from normal turbinates.

Polyps are smooth, pale gray, avascular, mobile, nontender, and accompany chronic allergy.

Palpate the Sinus Areas

Using your thumbs, press over the frontal sinuses below the eyebrows and over the maxillary sinuses below the cheekbones. Do not press directly on the eyeballs. The person should feel firm pressure but no pain.

Sinus areas are tender to palpation in people with chronic allergies and acute infection (sinusitis).

Inspect the Mouth

Lips

Inspect the lips for color, moisture, cracking, or lesions (Fig. 9.6). Black persons may have bluish lips, which is normal.

In light-skinned people circumoral pallor occurs with shock and anemia; cyanosis with hypoxemia and chilling; cherry red lips with carbon monoxide poisoning; acidosis from aspirin poisoning or ketoacidosis.

Cheilitis (perlèche)—cracking at the corners.

Herpes simplex, other lesions (Table 9.2, p. 104).

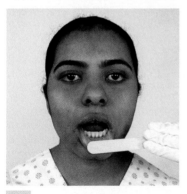

9.6

Teeth and Gums

Teeth normally appear white, straight, evenly spaced, and clean and free of debris or decay. Note any diseased, absent, loose, or abnormally positioned teeth.

Discolored teeth—appear brown with excessive fluoride use, yellow with tobacco use.

Grinding down of tooth surface. Plaque—Soft debris. Caries—Decay.

Normal Range of Findings	Abnormal Findings
Ask the person to bite and note alignment of the upper and lower jaw. Normal occlusion in the back is upper teeth resting directly on the lowers; in the front, the upper incisors slightly override the lower incisors.	Malocclusion, e.g., protrusion of upper or lower incisors.
Normally, the gums look pink or coral with a stippled (dotted) surface. Gum margins are tight and well defined. Check for swelling; retraction of gingival margins; and spongy, bleeding, or discolored gums. Black persons normally may have a dark, melanotic line along the gingival margin.	Gingival hypertrophy, crevices between teeth and gums, pockets of debris. Gums bleed with slight pressure, indicating gingivitis. Dark line on gingival margins occurs with lead and bismuth poisoning.

Tongue

The tongue color is pink and even. The dorsal surface is normally roughened from the papillae. A thin white coating may be present. Ask the person to touch the tongue to the roof of the mouth. Its ventral surface looks smooth and glistening and shows veins. Saliva is present.	Beefy red, swollen tongue. Smooth glossy areas (see Table 17.5, p. 373, in Jarvis: *Physical Examination and Health Assessment,* 8th ed.). Enlarged tongue occurs with mental retardation, hypothyroidism, acromegaly. Dry mouth occurs with dehydration, fever; tongue has deep vertical fissures.
With a glove, hold the tongue with a cotton gauze pad for traction and swing it out and to each side (Fig. 9.7). Inspect for any white patches or lesions—normally none are present. If any occur, palpate these lesions for induration.	Oral precancerous and cancerous lesions (see Table 17.5 in Jarvis: *Physical Examination and Health Assessment,* 8th ed.).

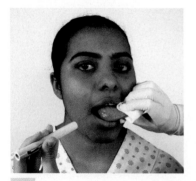

9.7

Normal Range of Findings	Abnormal Findings

Carefully inspect the tongue and the entire U-shaped area under the tongue. Note any white patches, nodules, or ulcerations. If lesions are present or with any person older than 50 years of age or with a positive history of smoking or alcohol use, palpate the area with a gloved hand. Notice any induration.

Excessive saliva and drooling.

Any lesion or ulcer persisting for more than 2 weeks must be investigated.

Indurated area may be a mass or lymphadenopathy and must be investigated.

Buccal Mucosa

The buccal mucosa looks pink, smooth, and moist, although patchy hyperpigmentation is common and normal in dark-skinned people.

Dappled brown patches are present with Addison disease (chronic adrenal insufficiency).

Stensen duct, the opening of the parotid salivary gland, looks like a small dimple opposite the upper second molar. You may also see a raised occlusion line on the buccal mucosa parallel with the level the teeth meet; this is due to the teeth closing against the cheek.

Orifice of Stensen duct looks red with mumps.

Koplik spots—Small blue-white spots are prodromal sign of measles.

Fordyce granules are small, isolated white or yellow papules on the mucosa of cheek, tongue, and lips. These little sebaceous cysts are painless and not significant.

The chalky white raised patch of *leukoplakia* is precancerous (see Table 17.4, p. 372, in Jarvis: *Physical Examination and Health Assessment,* 8th ed.).

Palate

The more anterior hard palate is white with irregular transverse rugae. The posterior soft palate is pink, smooth, and upwardly movable. A common variation is a nodular bony ridge down the middle of the hard palate, a **torus palatinus** (see Table 9.2).

The hard palate appears yellow with jaundice. In blacks with jaundice it may look yellow, muddy yellow, or green-brown.

Oral *Kaposi sarcoma* is a bruise-like, dark red, macular lesion, usually on the hard palate, that is a common early lesion with AIDS.

Ask the person to say "ahhh" and note the soft palate and uvula rise in the midline. This tests one function of cranial nerve X, the vagus nerve.

A *bifid* uvula appears as if split in two; it is more common in Native Americans (see Table 17.6, p. 374, in Jarvis: *Physical Examination and Health Assessment,* 8th ed.).

Inspect the Throat

The **tonsils** are the same pink as the oral mucosa, and their surface is peppered with indentations or crypts. There should be no exudate on the tonsils. Tonsils are graded in size as:

With an acute infection tonsils are bright red and swollen and may have exudate or large white spots. A white membrane covering the tonsils may accompany infectious mononucleosis, leukemia, and diphtheria.

Normal Range of Findings	Abnormal Findings
1+: Visible 2+: Halfway between tonsillar pillars and uvula 3+: Touching the uvula 4+: Touching each other You may normally see 1+ or 2+ tonsils in healthy people, especially in children.	Tonsils are enlarged to 2+, 3+, or 4+ with an acute infection.
Depress the tongue with a tongue blade. Scan the posterior pharyngeal wall for color, exudate, and lesions. When finished, discard the tongue blade.	
Test cranial nerve XII, the hypoglossal nerve, by asking the person to stick out the tongue. It should protrude in the midline. Children enjoy this request. Note any tremor, loss of movement, or deviation to the side.	With damage to cranial nerve XII, the tongue deviates toward the paralyzed side. A fine tremor of the tongue occurs with hyperthyroidism, a coarse tremor with cerebral palsy and alcoholism.
Notice any breath odor, *halitosis.* This is common and usually from a local cause such as poor oral hygiene, consumption of odoriferous foods, alcohol consumption, heavy smoking, or dental infection. Occasionally it may indicate a systemic disease.	Diabetic ketoacidosis has an accompanying sweet fruity breath odor; this acetone smell also occurs in children with malnutrition or dehydration. Others are an ammonia breath odor with uremia; a musty odor with liver disease; a foul, fetid odor with dental or respiratory infections; and alcohol odor with alcohol ingestion or chemicals.

❖ DEVELOPMENTAL COMPETENCE

Infants and Children

The newborn may have milia across the nose. The nasal bridge may be flat in black and Asian children. There should be no nasal flaring or narrowing with breathing.	Nasal flaring in the infant indicates respiratory distress. In a child with chronic allergy a transverse ridge is present across the nose from wiping the nose upward with the palm. Nasal narrowing on inhalation is seen with chronic nasal obstruction and mouth breathing.
Note the number of teeth and whether it is appropriate for the child's age. Also note patterns of eruption, position, condition, and hygiene. Use this guide for children younger than 2 years: the child's age in months minus the number 6 should equal the expected	No teeth by age 1 year. Discolored teeth—Appear yellow or yellow-brown with infants taking tetracycline or whose mothers took the drug during the last trimester; appear green or black with excessive iron ingestion, although this reverses when the iron is stopped.

Normal Range of Findings	Abnormal Findings
number of deciduous teeth. Normally all 20 deciduous teeth are in by $2\frac{1}{2}$ years.	Nursing bottle caries are brown and occur in upper front teeth from taking a bottle of milk, juice, or soda into bed.
	Malocclusion—Upper or lower dental arches are out of alignment.
Note any bruising or laceration on the buccal mucosa or gums of infant or young child.	Trauma may indicate child abuse resulting from forced feeding of bottle or spoon.

The Pregnant Woman

Gum hypertrophy (surface looks smooth, and stippling disappears) may occur normally at puberty or during pregnancy (pregnancy gingivitis).

The Aging Adult

In the edentulous person the mouth and lips fold in, giving a "pursestring" appearance. The teeth may look slightly yellowed, although the color is uniform. The teeth may look longer as the gum margins recede. Tooth surfaces look worn down or abraded.

The tongue looks smoother because of papillary atrophy. The aging adult's buccal mucosa is thinned and may look shinier, as though it were varnished.

Old dental work deteriorates, especially at the gum margins. The teeth loosen with bone resorption and may move with palpation.

HEALTH PROMOTION AND PATIENT TEACHING

Smoking is the world's leading cause of early death and disability; smoking cigarettes leads to at least 22 diseases, including 12 types of cancer, 6 types of heart and blood vessel disease, diabetes, chronic obstructive lung disease, pneumonia, and influenza (Carter, Abnet, & Feskanich, 2015). So it is imperative that you make an effort to teach at every patient encounter. At the very least, consider the Very Brief Advice on Smoking, which you can adapt to your work situation. [Ask] *"Do you smoke or use tobacco products? At what age did you start smoking? How many packs of cigarettes per day do you smoke?*

How many years have you smoked this amount?" [Advise] *"Smoking cigarettes leads to many heart and lung diseases and to many types of cancer. Stopping smoking is the very best thing you can do to improve your health. The best way to quit is a combination of behavioral support and medication. We have a local, friendly stop-smoking service. The people there are experts, and I can send you to them if you'd like."* (Van Schayck, Williams, & Barchilon, 2017) [Act] Refer the person to the stop-smoking service, or make a note in the person's record that you have advised and the person is not ready to quit.

Summary Checklist: Nose, Mouth, and Throat

Nose
1. **Inspect external nose:**
   Symmetry
   Deformity
   Lesions
2. **Palpate to test patency of each nostril**
3. **Inspect nasal cavity using nasal speculum:**
   Color and integrity of nasal mucosa
   Septum for deviation, perforation, or bleeding
   Turbinates, noting color, any exudate, swelling, or polyps

4. **Palpate the sinus areas for tenderness**

Mouth and Throat
1. **Inspect using penlight:**
   Lips, teeth and gums, tongue, buccal mucosa
      Color, intactness of structures, lesions
   Palate and uvula
      Integrity and mobility as person phonates
   Grade tonsils
   Pharyngeal wall
   Color, any exudate, or lesions
2. **Palpate mouth when indicated**

DOCUMENTATION

Sample Charting

SUBJECTIVE

Nose: No history of discharge, sinus problems, obstruction, epistaxis, or allergy. Colds 1-2/yr, mild. Fractured nose during high school sports, treated by MD.

Mouth and Throat: No pain, lesions, bleeding gums, toothache, dysphagia, or hoarseness. Occasional sore throat with colds. Tonsillectomy, age 8. Smokes cigarettes 1 PPD × 9 years. Alcohol-1-2 drinks socially, about 2×/month. Visits dentist annually, dental hygienist 2×/year, flosses daily. No dental appliance.

OBJECTIVE

Nose: Symmetric, no deformity or skin lesions. Nares patent. Mucosa pink; no discharge, lesions, or polyps; no septal deviation or perforation. Sinuses—no tenderness to palpation.

Mouth: Can clench teeth. Mucosa and gingivae pink, no masses or lesions. Teeth all present, straight, and in good repair. Tongue smooth, pink, no lesions, protrudes in midline, no tremor.

Throat: Mucosa pink, no lesions or exudate. Uvula rises in midline on phonation. Tonsils out.

ASSESSMENT

Structures intact and healthy

ABNORMAL FINDINGS

TABLE 9.1	Abnormalities of the Nose

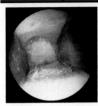

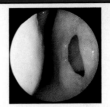

Foreign Body

Children particularly are apt to put an object up the nose (here, yellow plastic foam), producing unilateral mucopurulent drainage and foul odor. Because some risk for aspiration exists, removal should be prompt.

Perforated Septum

A hole in the septum, usually in the cartilaginous part, may be caused by snorting cocaine, chronic infection, trauma from continual picking of crusts, or nasal surgery. It is seen directly or as a spot of light when the penlight is directed into the other naris.

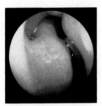

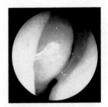

Acute Rhinitis (Nonallergic)

The first sign is a clear, watery discharge, rhinorrhea, which later becomes purulent. This is accompanied by sneezing and swollen mucosa, which causes nasal obstruction. Turbinates are dark red and swollen.

Allergic Rhinitis

Rhinorrhea, itching of nose and eyes, lacrimation, nasal congestion, and sneezing are present. Note serous edema and swelling of turbinates to fill the air space. Turbinates are usually pale (although they may appear violet), and their surface looks smooth and glistening. May be seasonal or perennial, depending on allergen.

TABLE 9.2	Abnormalities of the Mouth and Throat

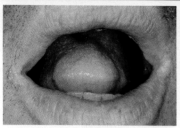

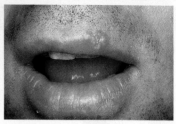

Cheilitis (Angular Stomatitis, Perlèche)

Erythema, scaling, shallow and painful fissures at the corners of the mouth occur with excess salivation and candidal infection. Seen in edentulous people and those with poorly fitting dentures that cause folding in of corners of mouth.

Herpes Simplex I (HSV-1)

Cold sores are groups of clear vesicles with a surrounding indurated erythematous base; evolve into pustules that rupture, weep, crust, and heal in 4 to 10 days. Likely site is the lip-skin junction. Recurrent herpes simplex may be precipitated by sunlight, fever, colds, allergy.

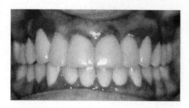

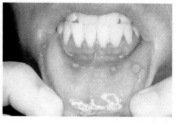

Gingivitis

Gum margins are red and swollen and bleed easily. Note bulbous gingivae between the teeth. Inflammation is usually due to poor dental hygiene or vitamin C deficiency. This may occur in pregnancy and puberty due to a change in hormonal balance.

Aphthous Ulcers

A canker sore appears first as a vesicle and then as a small, round ulcer with a white base surrounded by a red halo. It is quite painful and lasts for 1 to 2 weeks. The cause is unknown; it is associated with stress, fatigue, and food allergy.

Continued

TABLE 9.2	Abnormalities of the Mouth and Throat—cont'd

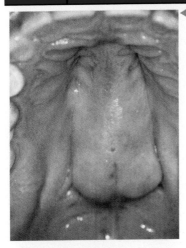

Torus Palatinus

A normal variation is a modular bony ridge down the middle of the hard palate (seen here using a mirror). This benign growth arises after puberty and is more common in Native Americans, Inuits, and Asians.

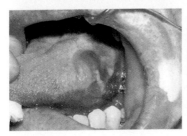

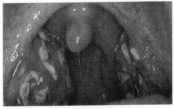

Carcinoma

An ulcer with rolled edges; indurated. Occurs particularly at sides, base, and under the tongue. It grows insidiously and may go unnoticed for months. It may have associated leukoplakia. Rich lymphatic drainage increases risk for early metastasis. Smoking and alcohol use account for most cases, and HPV-related oral pharyngeal cancers also are increased.

Acute Tonsillitis and Pharyngitis

Bright red throat; swollen tonsils; white or yellow exudate on tonsils and pharynx; swollen uvula; and enlarged, tender cervical and tonsillar nodes. Accompanied by severe sore throat, high fever of sudden onset. Most routine pharyngitis episodes are viral, resolve in 3-5 days. Severe symptoms lasting longer require throat culture or rapid antigen test to confirm streptococcal infection.

See Illustration Credits for source information.

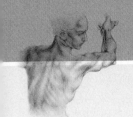

CHAPTER 10

Breasts, Axillae, and Regional Lymphatics

ANATOMY

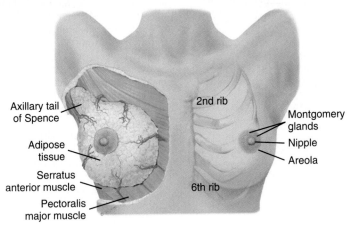

Axillary tail of Spence
Adipose tissue
Serratus anterior muscle
Pectoralis major muscle
2nd rib
Montgomery glands
Nipple
Areola
6th rib

10.1 Surface anatomy of the breast.

(© Pat Thomas, 2010.)

The female **breasts** are accessory reproductive organs whose function is to produce milk. The breasts lie anterior to the pectoralis major and serratus anterior muscles between the 2nd and 6th ribs (Fig. 10.1). The superior lateral corner of breast tissue, called the **axillary tail of Spence,** projects up and laterally into the axilla.

The breast may be divided into four quadrants by imaginary horizontal and vertical lines intersecting at the nipple. This makes a convenient map to describe clinical findings: upper outer quadrant, lower outer, lower inner, and upper inner.

Internally the breast is composed of (1) **glandular tissue,** which contains 15 to 20 lobes radiating from the nipple (Fig. 10.2). Each lobe empties into a lactiferous duct, and these converge toward the nipple. (2) The suspensory ligaments, or **Cooper ligaments,** are fibrous bands extending vertically from the surface to the chest wall muscles. They support the breast. (3) The **adipose,** or fatty, tissue provides most of the bulk of the breast.

The breast has extensive lymphatic drainage (Fig. 10.3): (1) **central axillary nodes,** high up in the middle of the axilla; (2) **pectoral** nodes, along the lateral edge of the pectoralis major muscle; (3) **subscapular** nodes, along the lateral edge of the scapula; and (4) **lateral** nodes, along the humerus, inside the upper arm. From the central axillary nodes, drainage flows up to the infraclavicular and supraclavicular nodes.

107

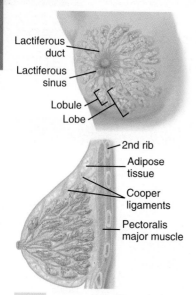

Lactiferous duct
Lactiferous sinus
Lobule
Lobe

2nd rib
Adipose tissue
Cooper ligaments
Pectoralis major muscle

10.2 Internal anatomy: (1) glandular tissue, (2) fibrous tissue including suspensory ligaments, (3) adipose tissue.
(© Pat Thomas, 2010.)

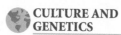

CULTURE AND GENETICS

Racial differences in sexual maturity show that African-American girls begin puberty about 1 to 1.5 years earlier and start menstruating about 8.5 months earlier than white girls (Herman-Giddens et al., 1997). Now into the 21st century the age of onset of breast development has dropped and is linked to the increase in body mass index (BMI) and the epidemic of obesity. Fat cells' aromatase secretes a form of estrogen that may account for the changes (Crocker et al., 2014). Current ages for onset of breast budding (Tanner stage 2) vary by race, ethnicity, and BMI: mean age of onset is 8.8 years for black girls, 9.2 years for Hispanic girls, 9.6 years for white girls, and 9.9 years for Asian girls. Overall, girls with greater BMIs achieved breast budding at younger ages (Biro et al., 2013). The obesity epidemic may be a "prime driver" in achieving early breast budding and then early menarche.

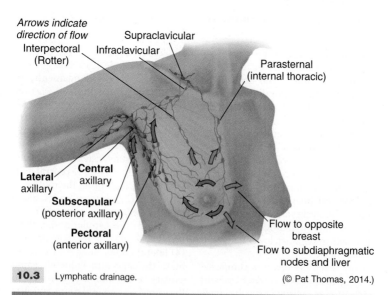

Arrows indicate direction of flow
Interpectoral (Rotter)
Supraclavicular
Infraclavicular
Parasternal (internal thoracic)

Lateral axillary
Central axillary
Subscapular (posterior axillary)
Pectoral (anterior axillary)

Flow to opposite breast
Flow to subdiaphragmatic nodes and liver

10.3 Lymphatic drainage.
(© Pat Thomas, 2014.)

SUBJECTIVE DATA

Breast
1. Pain
2. Lump
3. Discharge
4. Rash
5. Swelling
6. Trauma
7. History of breast disease
8. Surgery
9. Medications
10. Perform breast self-examination, last mammogram

Axilla
11. Tenderness
12. Lump or swelling
13. Rash

OBJECTIVE DATA

PREPARATION

The woman is sitting up, facing you. Use a short gown, open at the back, and lift it up to the woman's shoulders during inspection. During palpation the woman is supine; cover one breast with the gown while examining the other.

EQUIPMENT NEEDED

Small pillow
Ruler marked in centimeters
Pamphlet or teaching aid for breast self-examination

Normal Range of Findings	Abnormal Findings
Inspect The Breasts	
General Appearance	
Note symmetry of size and shape (common to have a slight asymmetry in size) (Fig. 10.4).	A sudden increase in size of one breast signifies trauma, inflammation, infection, or neoplasm.

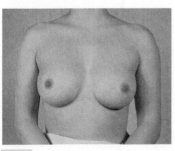

10.4 Breast appearance.

Normal Range of Findings	Abnormal Findings

Skin

The skin is normally smooth and of even color with no redness, bulging, dimpling, skin lesions, or focal vascular pattern. A fine blue vascular network normally is visible in lightly pigmented females during pregnancy. Pale linear striae, or stretch marks, often follow pregnancy.

Normally there is no edema.

Hyperpigmentation.

Redness and heat with inflammation.

Unilateral dilated superficial veins in a nonpregnant woman.

Edema exaggerates the hair follicles, giving a "pig skin" or "orange peel" look (also called *peau d'orange*).

Lymphatic Drainage Areas

The axillary and supraclavicular regions have no bulging, discoloration, or edema.

Nipple

The nipples should be symmetrically located and usually protrude, although some are flat and some inverted. Distinguish a recently retracted nipple from one that has been inverted for many years or since puberty.

Note any dry scaling, fissure or ulceration, and bleeding or other discharge. Normally there is none.

A normal variation in about 1% of men and women is *supernumerary nipple,* a congenital finding. Usually it is 5 to 6 cm below the breast near the midline and looks like a mole, although a close look reveals a tiny nipple and areola. It is not significant.

Deviation in pointing.

Recent nipple retraction signifies acquired disease (see Table 18.3, p. 398, in Jarvis: *Physical Examination and Health Assessment,* 8th ed.).

Any discharge must be explored, especially in the presence of a breast mass.

Rarely present, glandular tissue is a supernumerary breast or polymastia.

Maneuvers to Screen for Retraction

First ask the woman to lift her arms slowly over her head. Both breasts should move up symmetrically.

Next ask her to put her hands on her hips and push and then to push her two palms together. There will be a slight lifting of both breasts.

Retraction signs are due to fibrosis in the breast tissue, usually caused by growing neoplasms.

Note a lag in movement of one breast.

Note a dimpling or pucker that indicates skin retraction (see Table 18.3, p. 398, in Jarvis: *Physical Examination and Health Assessment,* 8th ed.).

Normal Range of Findings	Abnormal Findings

Inspect and Palpate the Axillae

Inspect the skin, noting any rash or infection. Lift the woman's arm and support it yourself so her muscles are loose and relaxed. Reach your fingers high into the axillae and move them firmly down in each direction (Fig. 10.5).

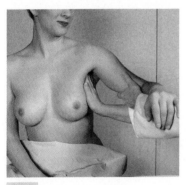

10.5

Usually nodes are not palpable, although you may feel a small, soft, nontender node in the central group. Expect some tenderness when palpating high in the axillae. Note any enlarged and tender lymph nodes.

Nodes enlarge with any local infection of the breast, arm, or hand and with the spread of breast cancer.

Palpate the Breasts

Help the woman into a supine position. Tuck a small pad under the side to be palpated and raise her arm over her head to flatten the breast tissue and displace it medially.

Normal Range of Findings	Abnormal Findings

Use the pads of your first three fingers and make a gentle rotary motion on the breast. For the vertical strip pattern (Fig. 10.6) start high in the axilla and palpate down the midaxillary to the bra line. Proceed medially in overlapping vertical lines ending at the sternal line. Vary your pressure so you are palpating light, medium, and deep tissue in each location. This should take you a few minutes with each breast.

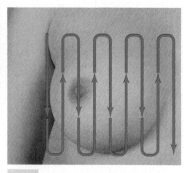

10.6   Vertical lines pattern of palpation.

In nulliparous women normal breast tissue feels firm, smooth, and elastic. After pregnancy the tissue feels softer and looser. Premenstrual engorgement is normal due to increasing progesterone and consists of a slight enlargement, a tenderness to palpation, and a generalized nodularity; the lobes feel prominent, and their margins are more distinct.

A firm transverse ridge of compressed tissue in the lower quadrants, the **inframammary ridge,** is especially noticeable in large breasts. Do not confuse it with an abnormal lump.

Heat, redness, and swelling in nonlactating and nonpostpartum breasts indicate inflammation.

Normal Range of Findings	Abnormal Findings

Palpate the nipple. Note any induration or subareolar masses. Use your thumb and forefinger to apply gentle pressure or a stripping action to the nipple. If any discharge appears, note its color and consistency. Pressing a white gauze pad to the discharge helps to determine its color.

Except in pregnancy and lactation, discharge is abnormal (see Table 18.6, p. 401, in Jarvis: *Physical Examination and Health Assessment*, 8th ed.).

If you feel a lump or mass, note these characteristics:

1. Location—Diagram the breast in the woman's record and mark the location of the lump
2. Size—In centimeters: width × length × thickness
3. Shape—Oval, round, lobulated, or indistinct
4. Consistency—Soft, firm, or hard
5. Movable—Freely movable or fixed
6. Distinctness—Solitary or multiple
7. Nipple—Displaced or retracted
8. Skin over the lump—Erythematous, dimpled, or retracted
9. Tenderness—To palpation
10. Lymphadenopathy

See Table 10.1 on p. 118 for description of common breast lumps using these characteristics.

HEALTH PROMOTION AND PATIENT TEACHING

Teach Breast Self-Examination (BSE)

Encourage the woman to become familiar with the look and feel of her breasts so she can detect any change and report it promptly. The best time to conduct BSE is right after the menstrual period or the 4th through 7th day of the menstrual cycle, when the breasts are the smallest and least congested. For the woman not menstruating (pregnant or menopausal), choose a familiar date as a reminder such as the first of the month.

Describe the correct technique, rationale, and expected findings (Fig. 10.7). At home she can start to palpate in the shower, where soap and water help palpation. Or she can lie supine. Encourage the woman to palpate her own breasts while you are there to monitor her technique.

Normal Range of Findings	Abnormal Findings

Breast Self-Examination

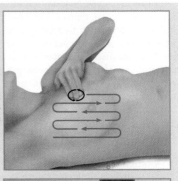

Lie down. Press the 3 middle fingers in a circular motion and use 3 levels of pressure. Follow an up-and-down pattern.

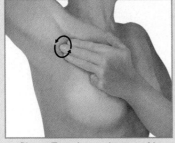

Sit up. Examine underarm with arm slightly raised.

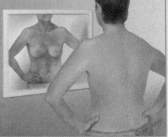

Note surface changes with hands pushed on hips, shoulders hunched.

10.7　　　　　　　　　　　　　　　　(© Pat Thomas, 2014.)

The Male Breast

Inspect the chest wall, noting the skin surface and any lumps or swelling. Palpate the nipple area for any lumps or tissue enlargement. It should feel even, with no nodules.

The normal male breast has a flat disk of undeveloped breast tissue beneath the nipple. **Gynecomastia** is an enlargement of this breast tissue, making it clinically distinguishable from the other tissue in the chest wall. It feels like a smooth, firm, movable disk. This occurs normally during puberty. It usually affects only one breast and is temporary.

Gynecomastia also occurs with use of some medications and in some disease states (see Table 18.8, p. 403, in Jarvis: *Physical Examination and Health Assessment,* 8th ed.).

Normal Range of Findings	Abnormal Findings

 ## DEVELOPMENTAL COMPETENCE

Infants and Children

In the neonate the breasts may be enlarged and secrete a clear or white fluid called *witch's milk*. These signs are not significant and are resolved within a few days to a few weeks.

The Adolescent

Adolescent breast development usually begins between 8 and 13 years of age. Expect some asymmetry during growth. Full development takes an average of 3 years, with a range of 1.5 to 6 years.

Note precocious development occurring before age 7 or 8. It occurs with thyroid dysfunction, stilbestrol ingestion, or ovarian or adrenal tumor.

Note delayed development occurring with hormonal failure, anorexia nervosa beginning before puberty, or severe malnutrition.

With the maturing adolescent, palpate the breasts as you would with the adult.

The breasts normally feel firm and uniform. Note any mass.

At this age a mass is usually a benign fibroadenoma or a cyst.

The Pregnant Woman

A delicate, blue vascular pattern is visible over the breasts of lightly pigmented females. The breasts increase in size, as do the nipples. Jagged linear stretch marks, or *striae,* may develop if the breasts have a marked increase in size. The nipples also become darker and more erect. The areolae widen, grow darker, and contain small, scattered, elevated Montgomery glands. On palpation the breasts feel more nodular, and thick yellow colostrum can be expressed after the first trimester.

The Lactating Woman

Colostrum changes to milk production around the 3rd postpartum day. At this time the breasts may become engorged; appear enlarged, reddened, and shiny; and feel warm and hard. Frequent nursing helps drain the ducts and sinuses and stimulates milk production.

Normal Range of Findings	Abnormal Findings
Nipple soreness is normal, appears around the twentieth feeding, lasts 24 to 48 hours, and then disappears rapidly. The nipples may look red and irritated and may even crack, but they heal rapidly if kept dry and exposed to air. Again, frequent nursing is the best treatment for nipple soreness.	One section of the breast surface appearing red and tender indicates a plugged duct (see Table 18.7, p. 402, in Jarvis: *Physical Examination and Health Assessment,* 8th ed.).

The Aging Woman

The breasts look pendulous, flattened, and sagging. Nipples may be retracted but can be pulled outward. The breasts feel more granular, and the terminal ducts around the nipple feel more prominent and stringy. Thickening of the inframammary ridge at the lower breast is normal and feels more prominent with age.	Because atrophy causes shrinkage of normal glandular tissue, cancer detection is somewhat easier. Any woman with a palpable lump not positively identified as a normal structure should be referred to a specialist.
Reinforce the value of BSE. Women older than 50 years of age have an increased risk of breast cancer (Table 10.2, p. 120).	

Summary Checklist: Breasts and Axillae

1. **Inspection:**
   Inspect breasts as woman sits, raises arms over head, pushes hands on hips, leans forward.
   Inspect supraclavicular and infraclavicular areas.

2. **Palpation:**
   Palpate axillae and regional lymph nodes.

   With woman supine, palpate breast tissue, including tail of Spence, nipples, and areolae.

3. **Teaching:**
   Teach BSE.

DOCUMENTATION

Sample Charting

FEMALE

SUBJECTIVE

States no breast pain, lump, discharge, rash, swelling, or trauma. No history of breast disease herself; does have mother with fibrocystic disease. No history of breast surgery. Never been pregnant. Performs BSE occasionally.

OBJECTIVE

Inspection: Breasts symmetric. Skin smooth with even color and no rash or lesions. Arm movement shows no dimpling or retractions. No nipple discharge, no lesions.

Palpation: Breast contour and consistency firm and homogeneous. No masses or tenderness. No lymphadenopathy.

ASSESSMENT

Healthy breast structure
Has knowledge of breast self-examination

MALE

SUBJECTIVE

No pain, lump, rash, or swelling.

OBJECTIVE

No masses or tenderness. No lymphadenopathy.

ABNORMAL FINDINGS

TABLE 10.1	Breast Lump

Benign Breast Disease

(Fibrocystic breast disease) Multiple tender masses that occur with numerous symptoms and physical findings: (1) Swelling and tenderness (cyclic discomfort); (2) Nodularity (significant lumpiness, both cyclic and noncyclic); (3) Dominant lumps (including cysts and fibroadenomas); (4) Nipple discharge (including intraductal papilloma and duct ectasia); (5) Infections and inflammations (including subareolar abscess, lactational mastitis, breast abscess, and Mondor disease)

Many women have some form of benign breast disease. Nodularity occurs bilaterally; nodules are regular, firm, mobile, well demarcated, and rubbery, like small water balloons. Pain may be dull, heavy, and cyclic or may occur just before menses as nodules enlarge. Some women have nodularity but no pain. Cysts are discrete, fluid-filled sacs. Dominant lumps and nipple discharge must be investigated carefully and may need to undergo biopsy to rule out cancer. Nodularity itself is not premalignant, but produces difficulty in detecting other cancerous lumps.

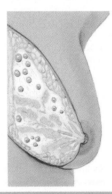

Continued

TABLE 10.1	Breast Lump—cont'd

Cancer

Solitary, unilateral, 3-dimensional, usually nontender mass. Solid, hard, dense, and fixed to underlying tissues or skin as cancer becomes invasive. Borders are irregular and poorly delineated. Grows constantly. Most common in upper outer quadrant. Usually found in women ages 30 to 80 years; increased risk across all ages until 80 years. As cancer advances, signs include firm or hard irregular axillary nodes, skin dimpling, nipple retraction, elevation, and discharge.

Fibroadenoma

Benign mass, most commonly self-detected in late adolescence and early adulthood. Solitary nontender mass that is solid, firm, rubbery and elastic. Round, oval or lobulated; 1 to 5 cm. Freely movable, slippery, fingers slide it easily through tissue. Usually no axillary lymphadenopathy but frequently painful. Diagnose by palpation, ultrasound, and needle biopsy.

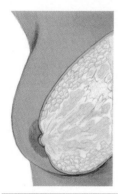
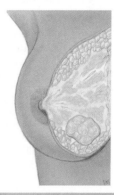

TABLE 10.2	Breast Cancer Risk Factors in Women[a]
Relative Risk	**Factor**
>4.0	• Age (65+ vs. <65 years, although risk increases across all ages until age 80) • Biopsy-confirmed atypical hyperplasia • Certain inherited genetic mutations for breast cancer (*BRCA1* and/or *BRCA2*) • Ductal carcinoma in situ • Lobular carcinoma in situ • Mammographically dense breasts • Personal history of early-onset (<40 years) breast cancer • Two or more first-degree relatives with breast cancer diagnosed at an early age
2.1-4.0	• Personal history of breast cancer (40+ years) • High endogenous estrogen or testosterone levels (postmenopausal) • High-dose radiation to chest • One first-degree relative with breast cancer
1.1-2.0	• Alcohol consumption • Ashkenazi Jewish heritage • Diethylstilbestrol (DES) exposure • Early menarche (<12 years) • Height (tall) • High socioeconomic status • Late age at first full-term pregnancy (>30 years) • Late menopause (>55 years) • Never breastfed a child • No full-term pregnancies • Obesity (postmenopausal)/adult weight gain • Personal history of endometrial, ovarian, or colon cancer • Proliferative breast disease without atypia (ductal) hyperplasia and fibroadenoma • Recent and long-term use of menopausal hormone therapy containing estrogen and progestin • Recent oral contraceptive use

From American Cancer Society (2018). *Breast Cancer Facts & Figures 2017-2018*. Atlanta: American Cancer Society.
[a]Relative risk compares the risk of disease among people with a particular exposure to the risk to the risk among people without that exposure. If the relative risk is above 1.0, risk is higher among exposed than unexposed persons.

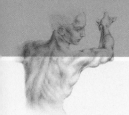

CHAPTER 11

Thorax and Lungs

ANATOMY

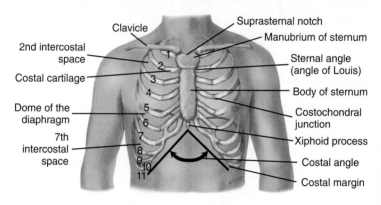

ANTERIOR THORACIC CAGE

11.1 Surface landmarks of the thoracic cage.   (© Pat Thomas, 2010.)

The **thoracic cage** is a bony structure with a conical shape (Fig. 11.1). It is defined by the sternum, 12 pairs of ribs, 12 thoracic vertebrae, and the diaphragm.

The *costochondral junctions* are the points at which the ribs join their cartilages. They are not palpable.

The *suprasternal notch* is the hollow U-shaped depression just above the sternum, between the clavicles.

The *sternal angle,* or angle of Louis, is the articulation of the manubrium and body of the sternum. It marks the site of tracheal bifurcation is continuous with the 2nd rib. Each

intercostal space is numbered by the rib above it.

The *costal angle* is formed by the right and left costal margins where they meet at the xiphoid process. It is usually 90 degrees or less.

The **trachea** lies anterior to the esophagus and is 10 to 11 cm long in adults (Fig. 11.2). It begins at the level of the cricoid cartilage in the neck and bifurcates just below the sternal angle into the right and left main bronchi.

An **acinus** is a functional respiratory unit and consists of the bronchioles and alveoli. Gaseous exchange occurs across the respiratory membrane

121

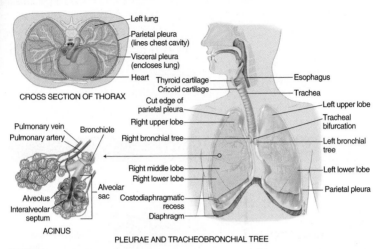

CROSS SECTION OF THORAX

Left lung
Parietal pleura (lines chest cavity)
Visceral pleura (encloses lung)
Heart

Thyroid cartilage
Cricoid cartilage
Cut edge of parietal pleura
Right upper lobe
Right bronchial tree

Esophagus
Trachea
Left upper lobe
Tracheal bifurcation
Left bronchial tree

Pulmonary vein
Pulmonary artery
Bronchiole

Right middle lobe
Right lower lobe
Costodiaphragmatic recess
Diaphragm

Left lower lobe
Parietal pleura

Alveolus
Interalveolar septum
Alveolar sac

ACINUS

PLEURAE AND TRACHEOBRONCHIAL TREE

11.2 Trachea and bronchial tree.   (© Pat Thomas, 2010.)

in the alveolar duct and the millions of alveoli.

In the **anterior chest** the *apex*, or highest point, of lung tissue is 3 or 4 cm above the inner third of the clavicles (Fig. 11.3). The *base*, or lower border, rests on the diaphragm. The right lung has 3 lobes, and the left lung has 2 lobes. The lobes are separated by fissures.

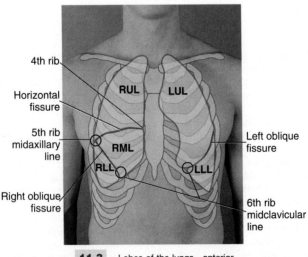

4th rib
Horizontal fissure
5th rib midaxillary line
Right oblique fissure

RUL   LUL
RML
RLL   LLL

Left oblique fissure
6th rib midclavicular line

11.3 Lobes of the lungs—anterior.

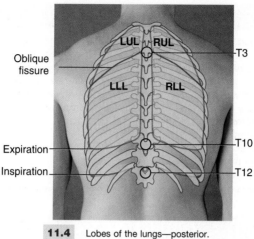

Oblique fissure

LUL RUL

LLL RLL

T3

Expiration

Inspiration

T10

T12

11.4 Lobes of the lungs—posterior.

Posteriorly the location of the 7th cervical vertebra (C7) marks the apex of lung tissue, and T10 usually corresponds to the base (Fig. 11.4). The most remarkable point about the posterior chest is that it is almost all lower lobe. The upper lobes occupy only a small band of tissue from the apices down to T3 or T4. The rest is all lower lobe. The right middle lobe does not project onto the posterior chest.

CULTURE AND GENETICS

Tobacco smoking causes almost 90% of **lung cancers,** and smoking causes a high mutational burden (Swanton & Govindan, 2016). This means that there are many mutations in the DNA genome of smokers compared with the very low mutation rate in nonsmokers. The complexity of this high mutation rate is what makes it so difficult to identify targeted drug treatments against lung cancer.

In the United States, the incidence of **tuberculosis** (TB) has declined slightly each year through 2016. Among U.S.-born persons, TB incidence is stable among Caucasians and Asians and has decreased in all other racial/ethnic groups, including Hispanics, African Americans, American Indian/Alaska Natives, and Native Hawaiian/Pacific Islanders (Schmit et al., 2017). However, almost 68% of U.S. cases occur among foreign-born persons; about 90% of these cases are attributable to reactivation of latent TB.

The prevalence of **asthma** is 8.4% in children ages <18 years, making it the most common chronic disease in childhood. The highest burden of asthma is among those living at or below the federal poverty level. By race/ethnicity, as of 2015 asthma prevalence has remained at 7.8% in white non-Hispanics and has decreased somewhat in black non-Hispanics (10.3%) and among Hispanics (6.6%) (CDC, 2017).

SUBJECTIVE DATA

1. Cough (duration, productive of sputum)
2. Shortness of breath (with level of activity)
3. Chest pain with breathing
4. Past history of respiratory disease (bronchitis, emphysema, asthma, pneumonia, tuberculosis)
5. Smoking history (age started, number of packs per day, number of years smoked)
6. Environmental exposure (e.g., home or occupational hazard, urban environment)
7. Patient-centered care (last TB skin test, chest x-ray image, influenza immunization)

OBJECTIVE DATA

PREPARATION

Ask the person to sit upright and males to disrobe to the waist. Leave the gown on females open at the back.

EQUIPMENT NEEDED

Stethoscope
Alcohol wipe (to clean endpiece)

Normal Range of Findings	Abnormal Findings
Inspect the Posterior Chest	
Shape and Configuration. The spinous processes are in a straight line. The thorax is symmetric with downward sloping ribs. The scapulae are placed symmetrically.	When severe, skeletal deformities, including scoliosis (S-shaped curvature) and kyphosis (outward curvature) of the thoracic spine, may limit thoracic cage expansion.
The anteroposterior (AP) diameter of the chest is less than the transverse diameter. The ratio of AP-to-transverse diameter is 1:2 or 0.7/1.	AP diameter that is equal to transverse diameter, or "barrel chest," with ribs horizontal, occurs in chronic emphysema due to hyperinflation of the lungs.
The neck muscles and trapezius muscles are developed normally for age and occupation.	Neck muscles are hypertrophied in chronic obstructive pulmonary disease (COPD) from aiding in forced respirations.
Position. This includes a relaxed posture with arms comfortably at the sides or hands in the lap.	With COPD, a tripod position (leaning forward with arms braced against knees, chair, or bed) gives leverage so the rectus abdominis, intercostal, and accessory neck muscles can aid in expiration.
Skin Color and Condition. Color should be consistent with person's genetic background, with no cyanosis or pallor. Note any lesions.	

Normal Range of Findings	Abnormal Findings

Palpate the Posterior Chest

Symmetric Expansion. Confirm *symmetric chest expansion* by placing your warmed hands on the postero-lateral chest wall with thumbs at the level of T9 or T10. Slide your hands medially to pinch up a small fold of skin between your thumbs. Ask the person to take a deep breath; your thumbs should move apart symmetrically. Note any lag in expansion.

Unequal chest expansion occurs with marked atelectasis or pneumonia, thoracic trauma such as fractured ribs, or pneumothorax.

Pain accompanies deep breathing when the pleurae are inflamed.

Tactile Fremitus. *Tactile fremitus* is a palpable vibration. Use the palmar base (the ball) of the fingers of one hand and touch the person's chest while he or she repeats the words "ninety-nine" or "blue moon." Start over the lung apices and palpate from one side to another; the vibrations should feel the same in the corresponding area on each side. (Fig. 11.5).

Decreased fremitus occurs when anything obstructs transmission of vibrations, e.g., obstructed bronchus, pleural effusions or thickening, pneumothorax, emphysema.

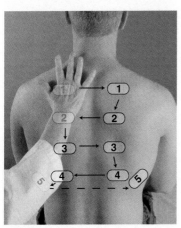

11.5

Normally fremitus is most prominent between the scapulae and around the sternum, sites where the major bronchi are closest to the chest wall. Fremitus normally decreases as you progress down because more and more tissue impedes sound transmission.

Increased fremitus occurs with compression or consolidation of lung tissue, e.g., lobar pneumonia (see Table 19.5, p. 436, in Jarvis: *Physical Examination and Health Assessment,* 8th ed.).

Normal Range of Findings	Abnormal Findings

Chest Wall. Using the fingers, gently *palpate the entire chest wall.* Note any areas of tenderness, increased skin temperature and moisture, any superficial lumps or masses, and any skin lesions.

Crepitus is a coarse, crackling sensation palpable over the skin surface. It occurs in subcutaneous emphysema when air escapes from the lung and enters the subcutaneous tissue, as after open thoracic injury or surgery.

Percuss the Posterior Chest

Lung Fields. Start at the apices and percuss in the interspaces: make a side-to-side comparison all the way down the lung region. Percuss at 5-cm intervals. Avoid the scapulae and ribs. **Resonance** predominates in healthy lung tissue in the adult. The resonant note may be modified somewhat in athletes with heavily muscular chest walls and in heavily obese adults in whom subcutaneous fat produces scattered dullness.[a]

Hyperresonance is found when too much air is present, as in emphysema or pneumothorax.

A **dull** note signals abnormal density in the lungs, as with pneumonia, pleural effusion, atelectasis, or tumor.

Auscultate the Posterior Chest

Breath Sounds. Instruct the person to breathe through the mouth a little bit deeper than usual. While standing behind the person, listen to the following lung areas—posterior from the apices at C7 to the bases (around T10) and laterally from the axillae down to the 7th or 8th rib. Use the side-to-side sequence illustrated in Fig. 11.6. You should expect to hear three types of normal breath sounds: **bronchial** (sometimes called *tracheal or tubular*), **bronchovesicular,** and **vesicular** (Table 11.1).

---

[a]The technique of measuring **diaphragmatic excursion** using percussion is no longer recommended for two reasons: (1) in persons with lung disease, evidence shows that clinicians usually overestimate diaphragmatic movement and that their results differ from chest image by 1 to 3 cm; and (2) evidence shows diaphragmatic excursion of <2 cm is an unreliable and infrequent sign of COPD (McGee, 2018).

Normal Range of Findings	Abnormal Findings

11.6 Order of auscultation.

TABLE 11.1	Characteristics of Normal Breath Sounds		
Type	Pitch	Duration	Normal Location
Bronchial (Tracheal)	High, loud	Inspiration < expiration	Trachea and larynx; sounds harsh, hollow, tubular
Bronchovesicular	Moderate	Inspiration = expiration	Over major bronchi where fewer alveoli are located: posterior, between scapulae, especially on right; anterior, around upper sternum in 1st and 2nd intercostal spaces
Vesicular	Low, soft	Inspiration > expiration	Over peripheral lung fields where air flows through smaller bronchioles and alveoli; sounds rustling like the sound of wind in the trees

Normal Range of Findings	Abnormal Findings
Note the normal location of the three types of breath sounds (Fig. 11.7; see also Fig. 11.8 on p. 130).	Decreased or absent breath sounds occur: 1. When the bronchial tree is obstructed by secretions, mucous plug, or a foreign body. 2. In emphysema due to loss of elasticity in the lung fibers and decreased force of inspired air. 3. When anything obstructs transmission of sound such as pleurisy or pleural thickening or air (pneumothorax) or fluid (pleural effusion) in the pleural space. **Increased breath sounds**—Bronchial sounds are abnormal over the peripheral lung fields. They occur when consolidation (e.g., in pneumonia) or compression yields a denser lung area that enhances the transmission of sound from the bronchi. When the inspired air reaches the alveoli, it hits solid lung tissue, which conducts sound more efficiently to the surface.

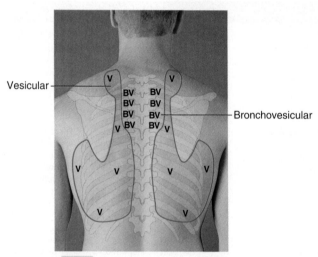

Vesicular

Bronchovesicular

11.7 Breath sounds on the posterior chest.

Adventitious Sounds. Note the presence of any **adventitious sounds.** These are abnormal sounds caused by

Normal Range of Findings	Abnormal Findings

the collision of moving air with secretions in the tracheobronchial passageways or by the popping open of a previously deflated airway.

Crackles (or rales) occur with pneumonia and pulmonary edema, and **wheezes** (or rhonchi) occur with asthma and emphysema (see Table 11.2 on p. 134).

Inspect the Anterior Chest

Shape and Configuration. The ribs are sloping downward with symmetric interspaces. The costal angle is within 90 degrees. Development of abdominal muscles is as expected for the person's age, weight, and athletic condition.

Barrel chest has horizontal ribs and costal angle greater than 90 degrees.
Hypertrophy of abdominal muscles occurs with chronic emphysema.

Facial Expression. Relaxed and benign, indicating an unconscious effort of breathing.

Level of Consciousness. Alert and cooperative.

Tense, strained, tired facies and pursed-lipped breathing accompany COPD.
Cerebral hypoxia presents with excessive drowsiness or anxiety, restlessness, and irritability.

Skin Color and Condition. The lips and nail beds are free of cyanosis or unusual pallor. The nails are of normal configuration.

Quality of Respirations. Normal, relaxed breathing is automatic and effortless, regular, and even and produces no noise. The chest expands symmetrically with each inspiration. Note any localized lag on inspiration.

Clubbing of fingertips occurs with chronic respiratory disease.
Noisy breathing occurs with severe asthma or chronic bronchitis.
Unequal chest expansion occurs when part of the lung is obstructed or collapsed, as with pneumonia, or with guarding to avoid postoperative incisional pain or the pain of pleurisy.
The rectus abdominis and internal intercostal muscles are used to force expiration in COPD.

The respiratory rate is within normal limits for the person's age, and the pattern of breathing is regular. Occasional sighs normally punctuate breathing.

Tachypnea and hyperventilation, bradypnea and hypoventilation, periodic breathing (see full description in Table 11.3 on p. 136).

Percuss the Anterior Chest

Begin at the apices. Percussing the interspaces and comparing one side to the other, move down the anterior chest.

Normally you hear a resonant note over healthy lung tissue. Note the borders of cardiac dullness normally found on the anterior chest and do

Lungs are hyperinflated with chronic emphysema, resulting in hyperresonance where cardiac dullness would be expected.

Normal Range of Findings	Abnormal Findings

not confuse these with suspected lung pathology. In the right hemithorax the upper border of liver dullness is located in the 5th intercostal space in the right midclavicular line. On the left, tympany is evident over the gastric space (see Fig. 19.24, p. 426, in Jarvis: *Physical Examination and Health Assessment*, 8th ed.).

Auscultate the Anterior Chest

Auscultate the lung fields over the anterior chest from the apices in the supraclavicular areas down to the 6th rib. Progress from side to side as you move downward and listen to one full respiration in each location.

You should expect to hear vesicular breath sounds over most of the anterior lung fields as indicated in Fig. 11.8.

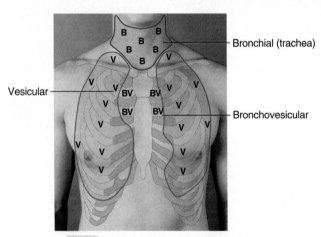

11.8   Breath sounds on the anterior chest.

DEVELOPMENTAL COMPETENCE

Infants and Children

Count the respiratory rate for 1 full minute when the infant is asleep, if possible, because infants reach rapid

Rapid respiratory rates accompany pneumonia, fever, pain, heart disease, and anemia.

Normal Range of Findings	Abnormal Findings

rates with very little excitation when awake (Fig. 11.9). The respiratory pattern may be irregular when there are extremes in room temperature or with feeding or sleeping. Brief periods of apnea less than 10 or 15 seconds are common. This periodic breathing is more common in premature infants.

In an infant tachypnea of 50 to 100 breaths/min during sleep may be an early sign of heart failure.

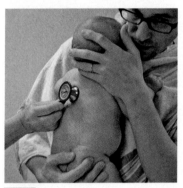

11.9

Auscultation normally yields bronchovesicular breath sounds in the peripheral lung fields in the infant and young child up to age 5 or 6 years because of the relatively thin chest wall with underdeveloped musculature.

Fine crackles are the adventitious sounds commonly heard in the immediate newborn period and are due to opening of the airways and clearing of fluid. Because the newborn's chest wall is so thin, transmission of sounds is enhanced and heard easily all over the chest, making localizations of breath sounds a problem. Even bowel sounds are heard easily in the chest. Try using the smaller pediatric diaphragm endpiece or place the bell over the infant's interspaces, not over the ribs.

Diminished breath sounds occur with pneumonia, atelectasis, pleural effusion, or pneumothorax.

Persistent fine crackles scattered over the chest occur with pneumonia, bronchiolitis, or atelectasis.

Crackles only in upper lung fields occur with cystic fibrosis; crackles only in lower lung fields occur with heart failure.

Expiratory wheezing occurs with asthma or bronchiolitis.

Persistent peristaltic sounds with diminished breath sounds on the same side may indicate diaphragmatic hernia.

Stridor is a high-pitched inspiratory crowing sound heard without the stethoscope that occurs with croup, acute epiglottitis, or foreign body aspiration.

Normal Range of Findings	Abnormal Findings

The Pregnant Woman

The thoracic cage may appear wider, and the costal angle may feel wider than in the nonpregnant state. Respirations may be deeper.

The Aging Adult

The chest cage commonly shows an increased anteroposterior diameter, giving a round barrel shape and **kyphosis** or an outward curvature of the thoracic spine. The person compensates by holding the head extended and tilted back.

You may palpate marked bony prominences because of decreased subcutaneous fat. Chest expansion may be somewhat decreased although still symmetric. The costal cartilages become calcified with age, resulting in a less mobile thorax.

An older person may tire easily, especially during auscultation when deep mouth-breathing is required. Take care that this person does not hyperventilate and become dizzy. Allow brief rest periods or quiet breathing. If the person does feel faint, holding the breath for a few seconds restores equilibrium.

Summary Checklist: Thorax and Lungs

1. **Inspection:**
   Thoracic cage
   Respirations
   Skin color and condition
   Person's position
   Facial expression
   Level of consciousness
2. **Palpation:**
   Confirm symmetric expansion
   Tactile fremitus

   Detect any lumps, masses, tenderness
3. **Percussion:**
   Percuss over lung fields
4. **Auscultation:**
   Assess normal breath sounds
   Note any abnormal breath sounds
   Note any adventitious sounds

DOCUMENTATION

Sample Charting

SUBJECTIVE

No cough, shortness of breath, or chest pain with breathing. No history of respiratory diseases. Has "one or no" colds per year. Has never smoked. Works in well-ventilated office on a smoke-free campus. Last TB skin test 4 years PTA, negative. Never had chest x-ray.

OBJECTIVE

Inspection: AP < transverse diameter. Respirations 16/min, relaxed and even.
Palpation: Chest expansion symmetric. Tactile fremitus equal bilaterally. No tenderness to palpation. No lumps or lesions.
Percussion: Resonant to percussion over lung fields.
Auscultation: Vesicular breath sounds clear over lung fields. No adventitious sounds.

ASSESSMENT

Intact thoracic structures
Lung sounds clear and equal bilaterally

ABNORMAL FINDINGS

TABLE 11.2	Adventitious Sounds[a]		
Sound	**Description**	**Mechanism**	**Clinical Example**
(1) Discontinuous Sounds			
Crackles—Fine (rales) Inspiration Expiration	Discontinuous, high-pitched, short, crackling, popping sounds heard during inspiration that are not cleared by coughing.	Inspiratory crackles: inhaled air collides with previously deflated airways; airways suddenly pop open, creating explosive crackling sound. Expiratory crackles: sudden airway closing.	*Late inspiratory crackles* occur with restrictive disease: pneumonia, heart failure, interstitial fibrosis. *Early inspiratory crackles* occur with obstructive disease: chronic bronchitis, asthma, emphysema.
Crackles—Coarse 	Loud, low-pitched, bubbling and gurgling sounds that start in early inspiration and in early expiration.	Inhaled air collides with secretions in the trachea and large bronchi.	Pulmonary edema, pneumonia, pulmonary fibrosis, and in end of life from a depressed cough reflex.
Atelectatic crackles 	Sound like fine crackles but do not last and are not pathologic. Disappear after the first few breaths. Heard in axillae and bases (usually dependent) of lungs.	When sections of alveoli are not fully aerated, they deflate and accumulate secretions. Crackles are heard when these sections reexpand with a few deep breaths.	In aging adults, bedridden persons, or people just roused from sleep.

[a]Although nothing in clinical practice seems to differ more than the nomenclature of adventitious sounds, most authorities concur on two categories: (1) discontinuous, discrete crackling sounds; and (2) continuous, musical sounds.

Continued

TABLE 11.2	Adventitious Sounds[a]—cont'd		
Sound	Description	Mechanism	Clinical Example
Pleural friction rub	A very superficial sound that is coarse and low pitched; it has a grating quality as if two pieces of leather are being rubbed together. Sounds just like crackles, but close to the ear.	Caused when pleurae become inflamed and lose their normal lubricating fluid. Their opposing, roughened pleural surfaces rub together during respiration.	Pleuritis accompanied by pain with breathing. (Rub disappears after a few days if pleural fluid accumulates and separates pleurae.)

(2) Continuous Sounds

Wheeze—High pitched (sibilant)	High-pitched, musical, squeaking sounds that predominate in expiration but may occur in both expiration and inspiration.	Air squeezed or compressed through passageways narrowed almost to closure by collapsing, swelling, secretions, tumors.	Obstructive lung disease such as asthma or emphysema.
Wheeze—Low pitched (sonorous rhonchi)	Low-pitched, musical snoring, moaning sounds. They are heard throughout the cycle, although they are more prominent on expiration. May clear somewhat by coughing.	Airflow obstruction. The pitch of the wheeze cannot be correlated to the size of the passageway that generates it.	Bronchitis.
Stridor	High-pitched, monophonic, inspiratory crowing sound; louder in neck than over chest wall.	Originates in larynx or upper airway obstruction from swollen, inflamed tissues or lodged foreign body.	Croup and acute epiglottitis in children and foreign body inhalation. Obstructed airway may be life threatening.

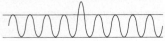

TABLE 11.3   Respiratory Patterns[a]

Inspiration Expiration

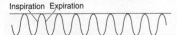

Normal Adult (for Comparison)
Rate—10 to 20 breaths/min
Depth—500 to 800 mL
Pattern—even
The ratio of pulse to respiration is fairly
   constant, about 4:1. Both values
   increase as a normal response to
   exercise, fear, or fever.

Sigh
Occasional sighs punctuate the normal
   breathing pattern and expand alveoli.
   Frequent sighs may indicate
   emotional dysfunction and may lead
   to hyperventilation and dizziness.

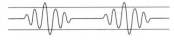

Tachypnea
Rapid shallow breathing. Increased rate
   >24 per minute. This is a normal
   response to fever, fear, or exercise.
   Rate also increases with respiratory
   insufficiency, pneumonia, alkalosis,
   pleurisy, and lesions in the pons.

Hyperventilation
Increase in both rate and depth.
   Normally occurs with extreme
   exertion, fear, or anxiety. Also occurs
   with diabetic ketoacidosis (Kussmaul
   respirations), hepatic coma, salicylate
   overdose, lesions of the midbrain,
   metabolic acidosis.

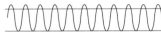

Bradypnea
Slow breathing. A decreased but regular
   rate (less than 10 breaths/min), as in
   drug-induced depression of the
   respiratory center in the medulla,
   increased intracranial pressure, and
   diabetic coma.

Hypoventilation
An irregular, shallow pattern caused by
   an overdose of opioids or anesthetics
   and with prolonged bedrest or
   conscious splinting of the chest to
   avoid respiratory pain.

Cheyne-Stokes Respiration
A cycle in which respirations gradually
   increase in rate and depth and then
   decrease. The breathing periods last 30
   to 45 seconds with periods of apnea (20
   seconds) alternating the cycle. Caused
   by severe heart failure, renal failure,
   meningitis, drug overdose, and
   increased intracranial pressure. Occurs
   normally in infants and older adults
   during sleep.

Biot Respiration
Similar to Cheyne-Stokes respiration
   except that pattern is irregular. A
   series of normal respirations (3 or 4)
   is followed by a period of apnea. The
   cycle length varies, lasting anywhere
   from 10 seconds to 1 minute. Seen
   with head trauma, brain abscess,
   heatstroke, spinal meningitis, and
   encephalitis.

[a]Assess the (1) rate, (2) depth (tidal volume), and (3) pattern.

CHAPTER 12

Heart and Neck Vessels

ANATOMY

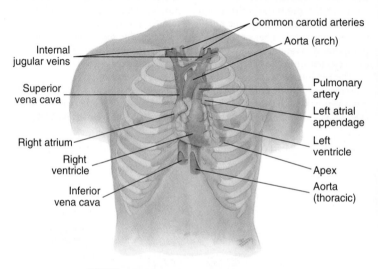

Internal jugular veins

Superior vena cava

Right atrium

Right ventricle

Inferior vena cava

Common carotid arteries

Aorta (arch)

Pulmonary artery

Left atrial appendage

Left ventricle

Apex

Aorta (thoracic)

12.1 Position of the heart and great vessels.

The **precordium** is the area on the anterior chest overlying the heart and great vessels. The heart extends from the 2nd to the 5th intercostal space and from the right border of the sternum to the left midclavicular line (Fig. 12.1).

Think of the heart as an upside-down triangle in the chest. The "top" of the heart is the broader **base,** and the bottom is the **apex,** which points down and to the left. During contraction the apex beats against the chest wall, producing an **apical impulse.**

The right side of the heart pumps blood into the lungs, and the left side of the heart simultaneously pumps blood into the body. Each side has an

atrium and a **ventricle** (Fig. 12.2). The atrium is a thin-walled reservoir for holding blood, and the thick-walled ventricle is the muscular pumping chamber.

There are four **valves** in the heart. The two **atrioventricular** (AV) valves separate the atria and the ventricles. The right AV valve is the **tricuspid;** the left AV valve is the **bicuspid,** or **mitral,** valve. The AV valves open during the heart's filling phase, or **diastole,** to allow the ventricles to fill with blood.

The **semilunar** (SL) valves are set between the ventricles and the arteries. They are the **pulmonic** valve in the right side of the heart and the **aortic** valve in the left side. They open during pumping, or **systole,** to allow blood to be ejected from the heart.

The **cardiac cycle** is the rhythmic movement of blood through the heart. It has two phases, **diastole** and **systole** (Fig. 12.3).

In **diastole** the ventricles relax and fill with blood. The AV valves, the tricuspid and mitral, are open. During the first rapid filling phase, **protodiastolic filling,** blood pours rapidly from the atria into the ventricles. Toward the end of diastole, the atria contract and push the last amount of blood into the ventricles, called **presystole.**

The closure of the AV valves contributes to the first heart sound (S_1) and signals the beginning of **systole.** The AV valves close to prevent any regurgitation of blood back up into the atria during contraction. Then the semilunar valves, the aortic and pulmonic, open, and blood is ejected rapidly into the arteries.

After the ventricles' contents are ejected, the semilunar valves close. This causes the second heart sound (S_2) and signals the end of systole.

Cardiovascular assessment includes the neck vessels—the carotid artery and the jugular veins (Fig. 12.4).

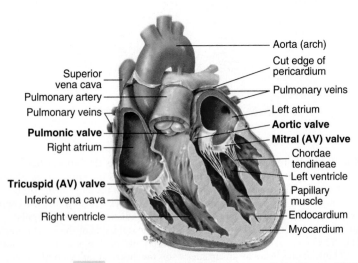

12.2   Heart wall, chambers, and valves.   (© Pat Thomas, 2006.)

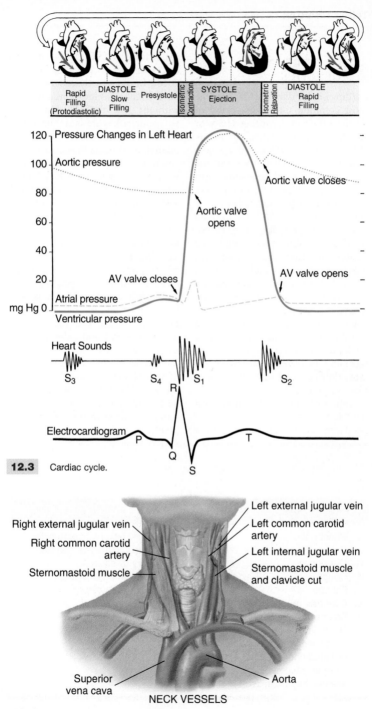

12.3 Cardiac cycle.

Pressure Changes in Left Heart

120 — Aortic pressure

Aortic valve closes

Aortic valve opens

AV valve closes

AV valve opens

Atrial pressure

mg Hg 0 — Ventricular pressure

Rapid Filling (Protodiastolic) · DIASTOLE Slow Filling · Presystole · Isometric Contraction · SYSTOLE Ejection · Isometric Relaxation · DIASTOLE Rapid Filling

Heart Sounds

S_3 S_4 S_1 S_2

Electrocardiogram   P   Q   R   S   T

NECK VESSELS

Right external jugular vein
Right common carotid artery
Sternomastoid muscle

Left external jugular vein
Left common carotid artery
Left internal jugular vein
Sternomastoid muscle and clavicle cut

Superior vena cava
Aorta

12.4 Neck vessels—the carotid artery and the jugular veins.

139

CULTURE AND GENETICS

Cardiovascular disease (CVD) is the most common underlying cause of death in the world, causing 31.5% of all global deaths (Benjamin et al., 2017). In the United States, the projections are that by 2030, 43.9% of the adult population will have some form of CVD. From 2004 to 2014, death rates attributable to CVD declined by 25.3% (Benjamin et al., 2017), but CVD data have a geographic difference. Recent national data show a lessening in the decline in heart disease mortality, especially in younger adults (Vaughan et al., 2017). Over 50% of U.S. counties showed increases in heart disease mortality among adults ages 35 to 64 years. These increases occurred in rural counties and in counties containing medium and small cities. Further, these mortality increases occurred at the same time as increases in obesity and diabetes prevalence.

Inherited DNA variation and lifestyle factors each contribute independently to the development of a major form of CVD, that of coronary artery disease (CAD) (Khera et al., 2016). In our genetic code, there are 50 different DNA locations associated with the risk of CAD, and a high polygenic risk score is significant for the risk of CAD events (myocardial infarction, coronary revascularization, and death). However, among persons with a high genetic risk, adopting a favorable lifestyle is associated with a 46% lower risk of CAD events than is an unfavorable lifestyle (Khera et al., 2016). A favorable lifestyle includes four healthy factors—no current smoking, no obesity (i.e., BMI <30), regular physical activity, and a healthy diet (i.e., fruits, nuts, vegetables, whole grains, fish, and dairy products, with lesser amounts of refined grains, processed meats, red meats, sugar drinks, trans fats, and sodium) (Khera et al., 2016). This evidence quantifies the interaction between genetics and lifestyle risk factors and shows that at every level of genetic risk, adopting a healthy lifestyle is associated with a significant drop in the risk of CAD events.

SUBJECTIVE DATA

1. Chest pain
2. Dyspnea
3. Orthopnea
4. Cough
5. Fatigue
6. Cyanosis or pallor
7. Edema
8. Nocturia
9. Past history (hypertension, elevated cholesterol, heart murmur, rheumatic fever, anemia, heart disease)
10. Family history (hypertension, obesity, diabetes, coronary artery disease)
11. Lifestyle (note: diet high in cholesterol, calories, or salt; smoking; alcohol use; drugs; amount of exercise)

OBJECTIVE DATA

PREPARATION

To evaluate the carotid arteries, the person may be sitting up. To assess the jugular veins and the precordium, the person should be supine with the head and chest slightly elevated. Stand on the person's right side.

EQUIPMENT NEEDED

Stethoscope with diaphragm and bell endpieces
Alcohol wipe (to clean endpieces)

Normal Range of Findings	Abnormal Findings

THE NECK VESSELS

Palpate the Carotid Artery

Gently palpate only one carotid artery at a time to avoid compromising arterial blood to the brain.

Feel the contour and amplitude of the pulse. Normally the contour is smooth with a brisk upstroke and slower downstroke, and the normal strength is moderate and equal bilaterally.

Diminished pulse feels small and weak (decreased stroke volume as in shock).

Increased pulse feels full and strong and occurs with hyperkinetic states (see Table 13.1, p. 165).

Auscultate the Carotid Artery

For people older than middle age or who show symptoms or signs of CVD, auscultate each carotid artery for the presence of a **bruit**. This is a blowing, swishing sound indicating blood flow turbulence; normally there is none.

Keep the neck in a neutral position. Lightly apply the bell of the stethoscope over the carotid artery at three levels: (1) the angle of the jaw, (2) the midcervical area, and (3) the base of the neck. Avoid compressing the artery because this could create an artificial bruit. Ask the person to hold his or her breath while you listen.

A bruit indicates turbulence from a local vascular cause, e.g., atherosclerotic narrowing.

A carotid bruit is audible when the lumen is occluded by $\frac{1}{2}$ to $\frac{2}{3}$. Bruit loudness increases as the atherosclerosis worsens until the lumen is occluded by $\frac{2}{3}$. When the lumen is completely occluded, the bruit disappears. Thus absence of a bruit could be an ominous sign of a completely occluded carotid lesion.

A **murmur** sounds much the same but is caused by a cardiac disorder. Some aortic valve murmurs radiate to the neck and must be distinguished from a local bruit.

Inspect the Jugular Venous Pulse

Position the person supine with the torso elevated anywhere from a 30- to a 45-degree angle. Remove the pillow

Normal Range of Findings	Abnormal Findings

to avoid flexing the neck. Stand on the patient's right, turn the head slightly away from the examined side, and direct a strong light tangentially onto the neck to highlight pulsations and shadows.

Note the external jugular veins overlying the sternomastoid muscle. In some people the veins are not visible at all; in others they are full in the supine position. As the person is raised to a sitting position, these external jugulars flatten and disappear, usually with bed at 45 degrees.

Unilateral distention of external jugular veins is from a local cause, e.g., kinking or aneurysm.

Fully distended external jugular veins above 45 degrees elevation show increased central venous pressure (CVP).

THE PRECORDIUM

Inspect the Anterior Chest

You may or may not see the **apical impulse**. When visible, it occupies the 4th or 5th intercostal space, at or inside the midclavicular line. It is easier to see in children or those with thin chest walls.

A **heave** or **lift** is a sustained forceful thrusting of the ventricle during systole. It occurs with ventricular hypertrophy and is seen at the sternal border or the apex.

Palpate the Apical Impulse

Localize the apical impulse precisely using one finger pad.
NOTE:
- Location—The apical impulse should occupy only one interspace, the 4th or 5th, and be at or medial to the midclavicular line
- Size—Normally 1 cm × 2 cm
- Amplitude—Normally a short, gentle tap
- Duration—Short, normally occupies only first half of systole

The apical impulse is palpable in about half of adults. It is not palpable in obese people or people with thick chest walls. With high cardiac output states (anxiety, fever, hyperthyroidism, anemia), the apical impulse increases in amplitude and duration.

Cardiac enlargement:
Left ventricular dilation (volume overload) displaces apical impulse down and to the left and increases size more than one space.

Increased force and duration but no change in location occurs with left ventricular hypertrophy and no dilation (pressure overload).

Apical impulse is not palpable with pulmonary emphysema due to hyperinflated lungs, which override the heart.

Normal Range of Findings	Abnormal Findings

Palpate Across the Precordium

Using the palmar aspects of your four fingers, gently palpate the apex, the left sternal border, and the base, searching for any other pulsations; normally there are none. If any are present, note the timing. Use the carotid artery pulsation as a guide or auscultate as you palpate.

A **thrill** is a palpable vibration. It feels like the throat of a purring cat. It signifies turbulent blood flow and accompanies loud murmurs. However, absence of a thrill does not necessarily rule out the presence of a murmur (see Table 12.2, p. 154).

Auscultate the Heart Sounds

Identify the auscultatory areas where you will listen. The four traditional valve "areas" (Fig. 12.5) are not over the actual anatomic locations of the valves but are the sites on the chest wall where sounds produced by the valves are best heard:
- Second right interspace—Aortic valve area
- Second left interspace—Pulmonic valve area
- Left lower sternal border—Tricuspid valve area
- Fifth interspace at around left midclavicular line—Mitral valve area

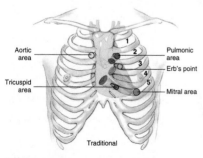
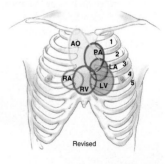

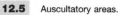

12.5   Auscultatory areas.

Do not limit your auscultation to only four locations because sounds produced by the valves may be heard all over the precordium. Learn to inch

Normal Range of Findings	Abnormal Findings

your stethoscope in a Z-pattern, from the base of the heart across and down and over to the apex; or start at the apex and work your way up. Include the sites shown in Fig. 12.5.

Begin with the diaphragm endpiece and clean it with an alcohol wipe. Use the following routine: (1) note the rate and rhythm; (2) identify S_1 and S_2; (3) assess S_1 and S_2 separately; (4) listen for extra heart sounds; and (5) listen for murmurs.

Note the Rate and Rhythm. The rate changes normally from 50 to 95 beats/min. The rhythm should be regular, although **sinus arrhythmia** occurs normally in young adults and children. With sinus arrhythmia the rhythm varies with the person's breathing, increasing at the peak of inspiration and slowing with expiration. Note any other irregular rhythm.

Premature beat—An isolated beat is early or a pattern occurs in which every 3rd or 4th beat sounds early.

Irregularly-irregular—No pattern to the sounds; beats come rapidly and at random intervals.

Identify S_1 and S_2. Usually you can identify S_1 instantly because you hear a pair of sounds close together ("lub-dup") and S_1 is the first of the pair. Other guidelines to distinguish S_1 from S_2 are as follows:

- S_1 is louder than S_2 at the apex; S_2 is louder than S_1 at the base.
- S_1 coincides with the carotid artery pulsation (Fig. 12.6).

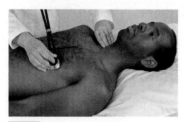

12.6

- S_1 coincides with the R wave (the upstroke of the QRS complex) if the person is on an ECG monitor.

Normal Range of Findings	Abnormal Findings

Listen to S_1 and S_2 Separately. Note whether each heart sound is normal, accentuated, diminished, or split. Inch your diaphragm across the chest as you do this.

Causes of accentuated or diminished **S_1** (see Table 20.4, p. 488, in Jarvis: *Physical Examination and Health Assessment,* 8th ed.).

Both heart sounds are diminished with increased air or tissue between the heart and your stethoscope such as emphysema (hyperinflated lungs), obesity, and pericardial fluid.

First Heart Sound (S_1). Caused by closure of the AV valves, S_1 signals the beginning of systole. You can hear it over the entire precordium, although it is loudest at the apex (Fig. 12.7).

S_1 S_2

| | APEX

LUB — dup

12.7

Second Heart Sound (S_2). S_2 is associated with closure of the semilunar valves. You can hear it with the diaphragm over the entire precordium, although it is loudest at the base (Fig. 12.8).

Accentuated or diminished **S_2** (see Table 20.5, p. 489, in Jarvis: *Physical Examination and Health Assessment,* 8th ed.).

S_1 S_2

| | BASE

lub — DUP

12.8

Splitting of S_2. A split S_2 is a normal phenomenon that occurs toward the end of inspiration in some people. Recall that closure of the aortic and pulmonic valves is nearly synchronous. Because of the effects of respiration on the heart, inspiration separates the timing of the two valves' closure, and the aortic valve closes 0.06 second before the pulmonic valve. Instead of one "DUP," you hear a split sound— "T-DUP" (Fig. 12.9). During expiration

Normal Range of Findings	Abnormal Findings

synchrony returns, and the aortic and pulmonic components fuse together. A split S_2 is heard only in the pulmonic valve area, the second left interspace.

SPLITTING OF THE SECOND HEART SOUND

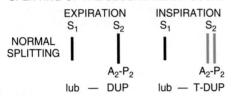

12.9

Concentrate on the split as you watch the person's chest rise up and down with breathing. The split S_2 occurs about every 4th heartbeat, fading in with inhalation and fading out with exhalation.

A *fixed split* is unaffected by respiration; the split is always there.

A *paradoxical split* is the opposite of what you would expect: the sounds fuse on inspiration and split on expiration (see Table 20.6, p. 489, in Jarvis: *Physical Examination and Health Assessment,* 8th ed.).

Focus on Systole, Then on Diastole, and Listen for Any Extra Heart Sounds. Listen with the diaphragm and then switch to the bell, covering all auscultatory areas. Usually these are silent periods. When you do detect an extra heart sound, listen carefully to note its timing and characteristics.

Listen for Murmurs. A murmur is a blowing, swooshing sound that occurs with turbulent blood flow in the heart or great vessels. Except for the innocent murmur described on the following page, murmurs are abnormal. If you hear a murmur, describe it by indicating these characteristics:

Timing. Systole or diastole.

Loudness. The intensity in terms of six grades:

• Grade 1—Barely audible, heard only in a quiet room and then with difficulty

During systole the **midsystolic click** is the most common extra sound. The S_3 and S_4 occur in diastole; either may be normal or abnormal (see Table 12.1, p. 152).

Conditions resulting in a murmur include (1) high rate of flow through a normal valve such as with exercise, pregnancy, or thyrotoxicosis; (2) restricted forward blood flow through a stenotic valve; (3) backward flow through a regurgitant valve; and (4) blood flow through abnormal openings in the chambers.

For a description of pathologic murmurs, using these characteristics, see Table 20.11, p. 496, in Jarvis: *Physical Examination and Health Assessment,* 8th ed.

Normal Range of Findings	Abnormal Findings

Normal Range of Findings

- Grade 2—Clearly audible but faint
- Grade 3—Moderately loud
- Grade 4—Loud; associated with a thrill palpable on the chest wall
- Grade 5—Very loud; heard with one edge of the stethoscope lifted off the chest wall
- Grade 6—Loudest; still heard with entire stethoscope lifted just off the chest wall

Pitch. High, medium, or low.

Pattern. Growing louder (crescendo), tapering off (decrescendo), or increasing to a peak and then decreasing (crescendo-decrescendo, or diamond-shaped). Since the entire murmur is just milliseconds long, it takes practice to diagnose pattern.

Quality. Musical, blowing, harsh, or rumbling.

Location. Area of maximum intensity of the murmur (where it is best heard) as noted by the valve area or intercostal spaces.

Radiation. Heard in another place on the precordium, the neck, the back, or the axilla.

Posture. Murmurs may disappear or be enhanced by a change in position.

Innocent Murmurs. Some murmurs are common in healthy children or adolescents and are termed **innocent** or **functional.** The contractile force of the heart is greater in children. This increases blood flow velocity. The increased velocity, plus a smaller chest measurement, makes an audible murmur.

The innocent murmur is generally soft (grade 2), midsystolic, short, and crescendo-decrescendo, with a vibratory or musical quality ("vooot" sound like fiddle strings). Also, the innocent murmur is heard at the 2nd or 3rd left intercostal space and disappears with sitting, and the young person has no associated signs of cardiac dysfunction.

Abnormal Findings

Although it is important to distinguish innocent murmurs from pathologic ones, it is best to suspect all murmurs as pathologic until proved otherwise. Diagnostic tests such as ECG and echocardiography are needed to establish an accurate diagnosis.

Normal Range of Findings	Abnormal Findings
Change Position. After auscultating in the supine position, roll the person toward his or her left side. Listen with the bell at the apex for the presence of any diastolic filling sounds.	S_3 and S_4 and the murmur of mitral stenosis may sometimes be heard only when on the left side.

DEVELOPMENTAL COMPETENCE

Infants

Auscultate with the small (pediatric size) diaphragm and bell. The heart rate may range from 100 to 180 beats/min immediately after birth and stabilize to an average of 120 to 140 beats/min. Infants normally have wide fluctuations with activity, from 170 beats/min or more with crying or being active to 70 to 90 beats/min with sleeping.

Expect the heart rhythm to have sinus arrhythmia, the phasic speeding up or slowing down with the respiratory cycle.

Rapid rates make it more challenging to evaluate heart sounds. Expect heart sounds to be louder in infants than in adults because of the infant's thinner chest wall. Splitting of S_2 just after the height of inspiration is common, not at birth, but beginning a few hours after birth.

Murmurs in the immediate newborn period do not necessarily indicate congenital heart disease. They are relatively common in the first 2 to 3 days because of fetal shunt closure. These murmurs are usually grades 1 or 2, are systolic, accompany no other signs of cardiac disease, and disappear in 2 to 3 days. The murmur of patent ductus arteriosus (PDA) is a continuous machinery murmur, which disappears by 2 to 3 days.

On the other hand, absence of a murmur in the immediate newborn period does not ensure a perfect heart; congenital defects can be present that are not signaled by an early murmur.

Persistent tachycardia:
- >200 beats/min in newborns or
- >150 beats/min in infants

Bradycardia:
- <90 beats/min

All warrant further investigation.

Investigate any irregularity except sinus arrhythmia.

Fixed split S_2 occurs with the murmur of atrial septal defect (ASD).

Persistent murmur after 2 to 3 days, holosystolic murmurs, diastolic murmurs, and those that are loud all warrant further evaluation.

For more information on murmurs due to congenital heart defects, see Table 20.10, p. 494, in Jarvis: *Physical Examination and Health Assessment,* 8th ed.

Normal Range of Findings	Abnormal Findings
It is best to listen frequently and to note and describe any murmur according to the characteristics listed on pp. 146-147.	

Children

Note any extracardiac or cardiac signs that may indicate heart disease: normally there are none.

The apical impulse is sometimes visible in children with thin chest walls.

Palpate the apical impulse in the 4th intercostal space to the left of the midclavicular line until age 4; at the 4th interspace at the midclavicular line from ages 4 to 6; and in the 5th interspace to the right of the midclavicular line at age 7.

The average heart rate slows as the child grows older, although it still varies with rest or activity.

The heart rhythm remains characterized by sinus arrhythmia. Physiologic S_3 is common in children (see Table 12.1). It occurs in early diastole, just after S_2, and is a dull, soft sound best heard at the apex.

Heart murmurs that are innocent (or functional) in origin are common throughout childhood. Most innocent murmurs have these characteristics: soft, relatively short systolic ejection murmur; medium pitch; vibratory; and best heard at the left lower sternal or midsternal border, with no radiation to the apex, base, or back.

Abnormal Findings:

Signs that indicate heart disease include poor weight gain, developmental delay, persistent tachycardia, tachypnea, dyspnea on exertion, cyanosis, and clubbing. Clubbing of fingers and toes does not appear until late in the first year, even with severe cyanotic defects.

Note any obvious bulge or any heave; these are not normal.

The apical impulse moves laterally with cardiac enlargement.

Thrill (a palpable vibration).

The Pregnant Woman

The vital signs usually yield an increase in resting pulse rate of 10 to 20 beats/min and a drop in BP from the normal prepregnancy level. BP decreases to its lowest point during

Normal Range of Findings	Abnormal Findings
the second trimester and then slowly rises during the third trimester. It varies with position. It is usually lowest in the left lateral recumbent position, a bit higher when supine (except for some who experience hypotension when supine), and highest when sitting. Palpation of the apical impulse is higher and lateral compared to the normal position because the enlarging uterus elevates the diaphragm and displaces the heart up and to the left and rotates it on its long axis. Auscultation of the heart sounds shows these changes due to the increased blood volume and workload: exaggerated splitting of S_1, increased loudness of S_1, and a loud, easily heard S_3. A systolic ejection murmur is common; heard at the left sternal border; grade 1, 2, or 3 in intensity. A continuous murmur arising from breast vasculature is termed the *mammary souffle* (pronounced soó fəl), which occurs near term or during lactation.	Gestational hypertension is BP ≥140/90 mm Hg on 2 separate measures, without proteinuria, starting after the 20th week of pregnancy. This returns to baseline after delivery.

The Aging Adult

A gradual rise in systolic BP is common with aging; the diastolic BP stays fairly constant, with a resulting widening of pulse pressure. Some older adults experience **orthostatic hypotension,** a sudden drop in BP when rising to sit or stand.

The chest often increases in anteroposterior diameter with aging. This makes it harder to palpate the apical impulse and to hear the splitting of S_2. The S_4 often occurs in older people with no known cardiac disease.

Occasional ectopic beats are common and do not necessarily indicate underlying heart disease. When in doubt, obtain an ECG; however, consider that the ECG records only one isolated minute and may need to be supplemented by 24-hour ambulatory heart monitoring.

Summary Checklist: Heart and Neck Vessels

Neck
1. **Carotid pulse:**
   Observe and palpate.
2. **Observe jugular venous pulse.**

Precordium
1. **Inspection and palpation:**
   Describe location of apical impulse.
   Note any heave (lift) or thrill.
2. **Auscultation:**
   Identify anatomic areas where you listen.

Note rate and rhythm of heartbeat.
Identify S_1 and S_2 and note any variation.
Listen in systole and diastole for any extra heart sounds.
Listen in systole and diastole for any murmurs.
Repeat sequence with bell of stethoscope.
Listen at the apex with person in left lateral position.

DOCUMENTATION

Sample Charting

SUBJECTIVE

No chest pain, dyspnea, orthopnea, cough, fatigue, or edema. No history of hypertension, abnormal blood tests, heart murmur, or rheumatic fever in self. Last ECG 2 yrs. PTA, result normal. No stress ECG or other heart tests.

Family history—Father with obesity, smoking, and hypertension, treated $\bar{c}$ diuretic medication. No other family history significant for CV disease.

Personal habits—Diet balanced in 4 food groups, 2 to 3 c. regular coffee/day; no smoking; alcohol, 1 to 2 beers occasionally on weekend; exercise, runs 2 miles, 3 to 4 ×/week; no prescription or OTC medications or street drugs.

OBJECTIVE

Neck: Carotid upstrokes are brisk and = bilaterally. No bruit. Internal jugular vein pulsations present when supine and disappear when elevated to a 45-degree position.
Precordium: Inspection. No visible pulsations; no heave or lift.
Palpation: Apical impulse in 5th ICS at left midclavicular line; no thrill.
Auscultation: Rate 68 bpm, rhythm regular, S_1-S_2 are crisp, not diminished or accentuated, no S_3, no S_4 or other extra sounds, no murmurs.

ASSESSMENT

Neck vessels healthy by inspection and auscultation
Heart sounds normal, no extra sounds

ABNORMAL FINDINGS

TABLE 12.1	**Diastolic Extra Sounds**

Third Heart Sound

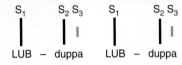

The S_3 is a ventricular filling sound. It occurs in early diastole during the rapid filling phase. Your hearing quickly accommodates to the S_3; thus it is best heard when you listen initially. It sounds after S_2, is a dull soft sound, and is low-pitched like "distant thunder." It is heard best in a quiet room, at the apex, with the bell held tightly (just enough to form a seal) and with the person in the left lateral position.

The S_3 can be confused with a split S_2.

Use these guidelines to distinguish the S_3:

Location—The S_3 is heard at the apex or lower left sternal border; the split S_2 is heard at the base.

Respiratory variation—The S_3 does not vary in timing with respirations; the split S_2 does.

Pitch—The S_3 is lower pitched; the pitch of the split S_2 stays the same.

The S_3 may be normal (physiologic) or abnormal (pathologic). The **physiologic S_3** is heard frequently in children and young adults; it occasionally may persist after age 40, especially in women. The normal S_3 usually disappears when the person sits up.

In adults the S_3 is usually abnormal. The **pathologic S_3** is also called a **ventricular gallop** or an **S_3 gallop,** and it persists when sitting up. The S_3 indicates decreased compliance of the ventricles, as in congestive heart failure. It may be the earliest sign of heart failure.

S_3 is also found in high cardiac output states in the absence of heart disease such as hyperthyroidism, anemia, and pregnancy. When the primary condition is corrected, the gallop disappears.

Continued

TABLE 12.1	Diastolic Extra Sounds—cont'd

Fourth Heart Sound

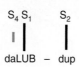

Pericardial Friction Rub

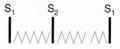

S₄ is a ventricular filling sound. It occurs when the atria contract late in diastole. It is heard immediately before S₁. This is a very soft sound, of very low pitch. You need a good bell, and you must listen for it. It is heard best at the apex, with the person in the left lateral position.

A **physiologic** S₄ may occur in adults older than 40 or 50 with no evidence of cardiovascular disease, especially after exercise.

A **pathologic** S₄ is termed an **atrial gallop** or an **S₄ gallop**. It occurs with decreased compliance of the ventricle such as in coronary artery disease and cardiomyopathy and with systolic overload (afterload), including outflow obstruction to the ventricle (aortic stenosis) and systemic hypertension.

Inflammation of the pericardium gives rise to a **friction rub**. The sound is high pitched and scratchy like sandpaper being rubbed. It is best heard with the diaphragm, with the person sitting up and leaning forward and with the breath held in expiration.

A friction rub can be heard any place on the precordium but is usually best heard at the apex and left lower sternal border, places where the pericardium comes in close contact with the chest wall. Timing may be systolic and diastolic.

The friction rub of pericarditis is common during the first week after a myocardial infarction and may last only a few hours.

TABLE 12.2	Abnormal Pulsations on the Precordium

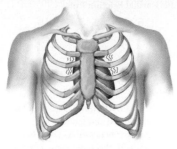

Base

A **thrill** in the second and third right interspaces occurs with severe aortic stenosis and systemic hypertension.

A thrill in the second and third left interspaces occurs with pulmonic stenosis and pulmonic hypertension.

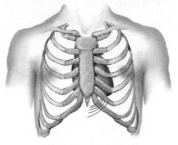

Left Sternal Border

A **lift** (**heave**) occurs with right ventricular hypertrophy, as in pulmonic valve disease, pulmonic hypertension, and chronic lung disease. You feel a diffuse lifting impulse during systole at the left lower sternal border. It may be associated with retraction at the apex because the left ventricle is rotated posteriorly by the enlarged right ventricle.

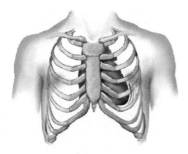

Apex

Cardiac enlargement displaces the apical impulse laterally and over a wider area when left ventricular hypertrophy and dilation are present. This is **volume overload**, as in heart failure, mitral regurgitation, aortic regurgitation, and left-to-right shunts.

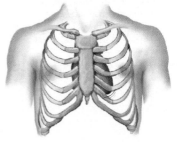

Apex

The apical impulse is increased in force and duration but is not necessarily displaced to the left when left ventricular hypertrophy occurs alone without dilation. This is **pressure overload**, as in aortic stenosis or systemic hypertension.

Images © Pat Thomas, 2006.

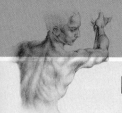

CHAPTER 13

Peripheral Vascular System and Lymphatic System

ANATOMY

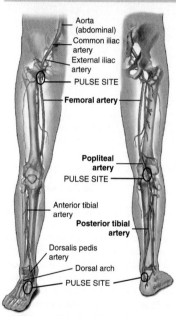

13.1 Arteries and pulse sites in the leg.
(© Pat Thomas, 2010.)

The **lymphatics** form a completely separate vessel system, which retrieves excess fluid and plasma proteins from the tissue spaces and returns them to the bloodstream. The lymphatic system also forms a major part of the immune system that defends the body against disease. Cervical lymph nodes drain the head and neck and are described in Chapter 6. Axillary lymph nodes drain the breast and upper arm and are described in Chapter 10.

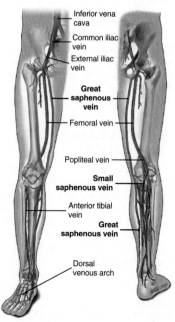

13.2 Veins in the leg.
(© Pat Thomas, 2010.)

The vascular system consists of the vessels in the body that transport fluid such as blood or lymph.

The heart pumps freshly oxygenated blood and nutrients through the **arteries** to all body tissues. The major artery to the leg is the **femoral artery**, passing down under the inguinal ligament (Fig. 13.1).

Veins drain the deoxygenated blood and waste products from the tissues and return it to the heart (Fig. 13.2).

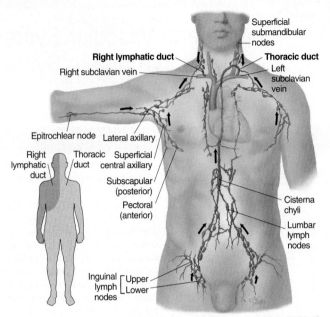

Superficial submandibular nodes

Right lymphatic duct

Right subclavian vein

Thoracic duct

Left subclavian vein

Epitrochlear node   Lateral axillary

Right lymphatic duct   Thoracic duct   Superficial central axillary

Subscapular (posterior)

Pectoral (anterior)

Cisterna chyli

Lumbar lymph nodes

Inguinal lymph nodes   ⌈Upper
⌊Lower

LYMPHATIC DUCTS AND DRAINAGE PATTERNS

13.3

(© Pat Thomas, 2010.)

The **epitrochlear** lymph node is in the antecubital fossa and drains the hand and lower arm (Fig. 13.3). The **inguinal** nodes in the groin drain most of the lymph of the lower extremity, the external genitalia, and the anterior abdominal wall.

🌎 CULTURE AND GENETICS

The prevalence of peripheral artery disease (PAD) increases dramatically with age; it is present in about 20% of people age 70 or older and 50% of people age 85 or older, and it is likely to increase, given the growing aging population (Chen et al., 2017). Only about 10% of people with PAD have the classic symptom of intermittent claudication (IC) (pain brought on by walking and relieved by rest) (Benjamin et al., 2017). Family history of PAD is independently and strongly associated with PAD prevalence and severity (Criqui & Aboyans, 2015). As for environmental factors, cigarette smoking is a particularly strong risk factor for all people with PAD, as are diabetes and hypertension. Other risk factors include elevated levels of total cholesterol and obesity (Criqui & Aboyans, 2015). Across the age ranges, African Americans have twice the burden of PAD compared with Caucasians (Carnethon et al., 2017). Traditional risk factors for African Americans are high (cigarette smoking, diabetes, hypertension), but adjusting for these does not eliminate the higher prevalence. Thus the health care team must provide comprehensive screening for African Americans, women, and all older adults, and tailor management of disease. The ankle-brachial index (ABI) is the first-line noninvasive test for PAD, and the technique is explained on p. 162.

SUBJECTIVE DATA

1. Leg pain or cramps
2. Skin changes on arms or legs
3. Swelling in legs
4. Lymph node enlargement (swollen glands)
5. Medications
6. Smoking history

OBJECTIVE DATA

PREPARATION

During a complete physical examination, examine the arms at the very beginning when you are checking the vital signs and the person is sitting. Examine the legs directly after the abdominal examination while the person is still supine. Then have the person stand up to evaluate the leg veins.

EQUIPMENT NEEDED (OCCASIONALLY)

Tape measure
Tourniquet or blood pressure cuff
Stethoscope
Doppler ultrasonic probe

Normal Range of Findings	Abnormal Findings
INSPECT AND PALPATE THE ARMS Note color of **skin** and nail beds; temperature, texture, and turgor of skin; and the presence of any lesions, edema, or clubbing, as described in Chapter 5. Check **capillary refill**. Depress and blanch the nail beds; release and note the time for color return. Usually the vessels refill within a fraction of a second. Consider it normal if the color returns in 1 or 2 seconds. Note conditions that can skew your findings, including a cool room, decreased body temperature, cigarette smoking, peripheral edema, and anemia. The two arms should be **symmetric** in size.	Refill lasting more than 1 or 2 seconds signifies vasoconstriction or decreased cardiac output (hypovolemia, heart failure, shock). The hands are cold, clammy, and pale. Edema of upper extremities occurs when lymphatic drainage is obstructed after breast surgery or radiation (see Table 21.2, p. 523, in Jarvis: *Physical Examination and Health Assessment,* 8th ed.).

Normal Range of Findings	Abnormal Findings

Note the presence of any scars on hands and arms. Many occur normally with usual childhood abrasions or with occupations involving hand tools.

Palpate both radial **pulses**, noting rate, rhythm, elasticity of vessel wall, and equal force. Grade the force (amplitude) on a three-point scale:

3+ increased, bounding
2+ **normal**
1+ weak
0   absent

Palpate the brachial pulses; their force should be equal bilaterally. Check the epitrochlear lymph nodes in the depression above and behind the medial condyle of the humerus.

Needle tracks in hands, arms, and antecubital fossae occur with intravenous drug use; linear scars in wrists may signify past self-inflicted injury.

Weak, thready pulse occurs with shock or peripheral arterial disease; full bounding pulse (3+) with hyperkinetic states (exercise, anxiety, fever), anemia, hyperthyroidism. Dropped beats; irregular pulse (see Table 13.1, pp. 165-166).

An enlarged epitrochlear node occurs with infection of hand or forearm, lymphoma, leukemia, infectious mononucleosis.

INSPECT AND PALPATE THE LEGS

Inspect both legs together, noting **skin** color, hair distribution, venous pattern, size (swelling or atrophy), and any skin lesions or ulcers.

Hair normally covers the legs. Even if leg hair is shaved, you will still note hair on the dorsa of the toes.

The **venous pattern** is normally flat and barely visible. Note obvious varicosities, although these are best assessed while the person is standing.

Both legs should be **symmetric in size** without swelling or atrophy. If the lower legs appear asymmetric, measure the calf circumference with a nonstretchable tape measure. Measure at the widest point, in exactly the same place, the same number of centimeters down from the patella or

Pallor with vasoconstriction; erythema with vasodilation; cyanosis.

Ulcers occur both with chronic arterial and chronic venous insufficiency (see Table 21.4, p. 525, in Jarvis: *Physical Examination and Health Assessment,* 8th ed.).

Malnutrition: thin, shiny, atrophic skin, thick-ridged nails, loss of hair, ulcers, gangrene.

Malnutrition, pallor, and coolness occur with arterial insufficiency.

Diffuse bilateral edema occurs with systemic illnesses, e.g., heart failure.

Unilateral swelling indicates a local obstruction, e.g., deep venous thrombosis (DVT), lymphedema.

Normal Range of Findings	Abnormal Findings

other landmark. Record your findings in centimeters.

Palpate for **temperature** along the legs and down to the feet, comparing symmetric spots. The skin should be warm and equal bilaterally. Bilateral cool feet may be due to environmental factors such as cool room temperature, apprehension, and cigarette smoking. If there is any increase in temperature up the leg, note whether it is gradual or abrupt.

A unilateral cool foot or leg occurs with arterial deficit.

Palpate the **inguinal lymph nodes**. It is not unusual to find palpable nodes that are small (1 cm or less), movable, and nontender.

Enlarged nodes, tender or fixed in area.

Palpate these **peripheral arteries** in both legs: femoral, popliteal, dorsalis pedis, and posterior tibial. Grade the force on the three-point scale.

Femoral Pulse. Locate the femoral arteries just below the inguinal ligament halfway between the pubis and anterior superior iliac spines (see Fig. 13.1). To help expose the femoral area, particularly in obese people, ask the person to bend his or her knees to the side in a froglike position. Press firmly and then slowly release, noting the pulse tap under your fingertips. If this pulse is weak or diminished, auscultate the site for a bruit.

A bruit occurs with turbulent blood flow, indicating arterial occlusion.

Popliteal Pulse. This is a more diffuse pulse and is hard to locate. With the person's leg extended but relaxed, anchor your thumbs on the knee and curl your fingers around into the fossa. Press your fingers forward hard to compress the artery against the bone. It is often just lateral to the medial tendon. A normal popliteal pulse is often impossible to palpate.

Posterior Tibial Pulse. Curve your fingers around the medial malleolus (Fig. 13.4). You will feel the tapping right behind it in the groove between the malleolus and the Achilles tendon.

The posterior tibial pulse and the dorsalis pedis pulse are diminished or absent in PAD.

Normal Range of Findings	Abnormal Findings

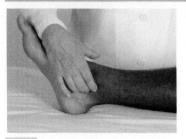

13.4 Posterior tibial pulse.

Dorsalis Pedis Pulse. This requires a very light touch. It is normally just lateral to and parallel with the extensor tendon of the big toe (Fig. 13.5).

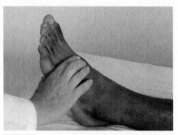

13.5 Dorsalis pedis pulse.

Check for pretibial edema. Firmly depress the skin over the tibia or the medial malleolus for 5 seconds and release. Your finger should normally leave no indentation, although a pit is commonly seen if the person has been standing all day or is pregnant. If pitting edema is present, grade it on this scale:

1+ Mild pitting; slight indentation; no perceptible swelling of the leg
2+ Moderate pitting; indentation subsides rapidly
3+ Deep pitting; indentation remains for a short time; leg looks swollen
4+ Very deep pitting; indentation lasts a long time; leg is grossly swollen and distorted

This scale is subjective.

Bilateral, dependent, pitting edema occurs with heart failure and hepatic cirrhosis.

Unilateral edema occurs with occlusion of a deep vein and unilaterally or bilaterally with lymphatic obstruction. With these factors, it is "brawny" or nonpitting and feels hard to the touch.

Normal Range of Findings	Abnormal Findings
Ask the person to stand so you can assess the venous system. Note any visible, dilated, or tortuous veins.	Varicosities occur in the saphenous veins (see Table 21.5, p. 526, in Jarvis: *Physical Examination and Health Assessment,* 8th ed.).

ADDITIONAL TECHNIQUES

The Doppler Ultrasonic Probe. Use this device to detect a weak peripheral pulse, monitor BP in infants and children, and measure a low BP or BP in a lower extremity (Fig. 13.6). The Doppler probe magnifies pulsatile sounds from the heart and blood vessels. Place a drop of coupling gel on the end of the handheld transducer. Place the transducer over a pulse site, tilted at a 45-degree angle. Apply very light pressure; locate the pulse site by the swishing, whooshing sound.

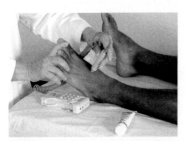

13.6   Using the Doppler to locate a pulse.

The Ankle-Brachial Index (ABI). The patient is lying flat with the head and heels fully supported (AHA, 2012). Confirm no smoking within 2 hours of the measurement and allow a 5- to 10-minute rest period supine before measurement. Choose the correct cuff width for the arm and the ankle; width should be 40% of limb circumference. Position the ankle cuff just above the malleoli with straight wrapping.

Normal Range of Findings	Abnormal Findings
Use the Doppler probe for both brachial and ankle measurements. In all sites locate the pulse by Doppler, inflate the cuff 20 mm Hg above disappearance of flow signal, then deflate slowly to detect reappearance of flow signal (AHA, 2012). Moving counterclockwise, measure: right arm, right posterior tibial (PT), right dorsalis pedis (DP), left PT, left DP, left arm. Calculate both ABIs using this formula:	AN ABI between 0.91 and 1 is borderline cardiovascular risk (AHA, 2012). An ABI of 0.90 or less indicates PAD. 0.90 to 0.70—mild claudication 0.70 to 0.40—moderate-to-severe claudication 0.40 to 0.30—severe claudication, usually with rest pain, except in the presence of diabetic neuropathy <0.30—ischemia, with impending loss of tissue

$$\text{Right ABI} = \frac{\text{Highest right ankle pressure (DP or PT)}}{\text{Highest arm pressure (right or left)}}$$

$$\text{Example:} \quad \frac{132\ \text{ankle systolic}}{124\ \text{arm systolic}} = \frac{1.06\ \text{or}\ 106\%, \text{indicating}}{\text{no flow reduction}}$$

$$\text{Left ABI} = \frac{\text{Highest left ankle pressure (DP or PT)}}{\text{Highest arm pressure (right or left)}}$$

See Jarvis, *Lab Manual for Physical Examination and Health Assessment,* 8th ed, Ch. 21, p. 188, for a grid format to record your findings.

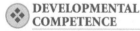

DEVELOPMENTAL COMPETENCE

Infants and Children

Transient acrocyanosis (i.e., symmetric cyanosis of the hands and wrists, feet, and ankles) and skin mottling may occur at birth. Pulse force should be normal and symmetric. Pulse force should also be the same in the upper and lower extremities.

Palpable lymph nodes occur often in normal infants and children. They are small, firm (shotty), mobile, and nontender. They may be the sequelae

Weak pulses occur with vasoconstriction, diminished cardiac output.

Full, bounding pulses occur with patent ductus arteriosus due to left-to-right shunt.

Diminished or absent femoral pulses and normal upper extremity pulses suggest coarctation of aorta.

Normal Range of Findings	Abnormal Findings
of past infection, e.g., inguinal nodes from a diaper rash or cervical nodes from a respiratory infection. Vaccinations can also produce local lymphadenopathy. Note characteristics of any palpable nodes and whether they are local or generalized.	Enlarged, warm, tender nodes indicate current infection. Look for source of infection.

The Pregnant Woman

Expect diffuse, bilateral pitting edema in the lower extremities, especially at the end of the day and into the third trimester. Varicose veins in the legs are also common in the third trimester.

The Aging Adult

The dorsalis pedis and posterior tibial pulses may be harder to find. Trophic changes associated with arterial insufficiency (thin, shiny skin; thick-ridged nails; loss of hair on lower legs) also occur normally with aging.

HEALTH PROMOTION AND PATIENT TEACHING

We don't often think about our feet, but good foot care can prevent serious problems later on. First, check your feet often.

Look for red spots, sensitive areas, discoloration, cuts, blisters, and ingrown toenails. Use a mirror to check the bottoms of your feet. If you have diabetes, check your feet every day.

Wash your feet regularly, especially between your toes. Dry feet carefully after a shower or bath, gently sliding a towel between each toe.

Keep toenails trimmed straight across, filed at the edges.

Wear clean socks every day.

Second, keep the blood flowing to your feet. Walking is a great way to do this, or try these indoor exercises:

Sit down and rotate your ankles in one direction, then the other, or try writing the alphabet from A to Z!

If you cannot walk very far, put your feet up when sitting or lying down, stretching and wiggling the toes.

If sitting for a long time, stand up and move around every half hour or so.

If you find yourself crossing your legs when sitting, uncross them often.

Summary Checklist: Peripheral Vascular System and Lymphatic System

1. **Inspect arms:**
   Color and size
   Lesions
2. **Palpate pulses:**
   Radial
   Brachial
3. **Check epitrochlear node**
4. **Inspect legs:**
   Color and size
   Lesions
   Trophic skin changes

5. **Palpate temperature of feet and legs**
6. **Palpate inguinal nodes**
7. **Palpate pulses:**
   Femoral
   Popliteal
   Posterior tibial
   Dorsalis pedis

DOCUMENTATION

Sample Charting

SUBJECTIVE

No leg pain, no skin changes, no swelling or lymph node enlargement. No history of heart or vascular problems, diabetes, or obesity. Does not smoke. On no medications.

OBJECTIVE

Inspection: Extremities have pink-tan color without redness, cyanosis, or any skin lesions. Extremity size is symmetric without swelling or atrophy.
Palpation: Temperature is warm and = bilaterally. All pulses present, 2+ and = bilaterally. No lymphadenopathy.

ASSESSMENT

Healthy tissue
Effective tissue perfusion

ABNORMAL FINDINGS

TABLE 13.1	Variations in Arterial Pulse

Description	Associated With

Weak "Thready" Pulse—1+. Hard to palpate; need to search for it; may fade in and out; easily obliterated by pressure.

Decreased cardiac output; peripheral arterial disease; aortic valve stenosis.

Full, Bounding Pulse—3+. Easily palpable; pounds under your fingertips.

Hyperkinetic states (exercise, anxiety, fever), anemia, hyperthyroidism.

Water-Hammer (Corrigan) Pulse—3+. Greater than normal force; then collapses suddenly.

Aortic valve regurgitation; patent ductus arteriosus.

Pulsus Bigeminus. Rhythm is coupled, every other beat comes early, or normal beat is followed by premature beat. Force of premature beat is decreased due to shortened cardiac filling time.

Conduction disturbance, e.g., premature ventricular contraction, premature atrial contraction.

Pulsus Alternans. Rhythm is regular, but force varies with alternating beats of large and small amplitude.

When heart rate is normal, pulsus alternans occurs with severe left ventricular failure, which is due to ischemic heart disease, valvular heart disease, chronic hypertension, or cardiomyopathy.

Continued

TABLE 13.1	Variations in Arterial Pulse—cont'd
Description	Associated With

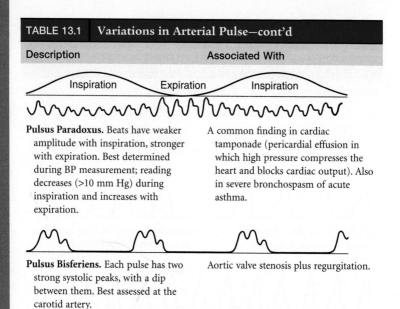

Pulsus Paradoxus. Beats have weaker amplitude with inspiration, stronger with expiration. Best determined during BP measurement; reading decreases (>10 mm Hg) during inspiration and increases with expiration.

A common finding in cardiac tamponade (pericardial effusion in which high pressure compresses the heart and blocks cardiac output). Also in severe bronchospasm of acute asthma.

Pulsus Bisferiens. Each pulse has two strong systolic peaks, with a dip between them. Best assessed at the carotid artery.

Aortic valve stenosis plus regurgitation.

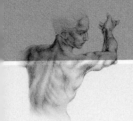

CHAPTER 14

Abdomen

ANATOMY

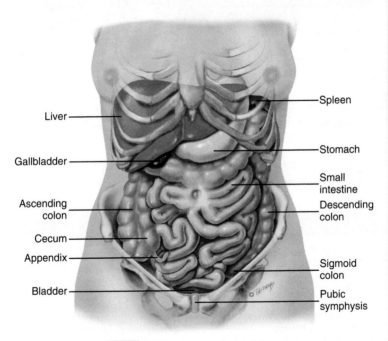

Liver

Gallbladder

Ascending colon

Cecum

Appendix

Bladder

Spleen

Stomach

Small intestine

Descending colon

Sigmoid colon

Pubic symphysis

14.1   Position of abdominal organs.   (© Pat Thomas, 2006.)

The **abdomen** is a large oval cavity extending from the diaphragm down to the brim of the pelvis (Fig. 14.1). For convenience in description, the abdominal wall is divided into four quadrants by imaginary vertical and horizontal lines bisecting the umbilicus.

The **aorta** is just to the left of midline in the upper abdomen (Fig.

14.2). At 2 cm below the umbilicus, it bifurcates into the right and left iliac arteries.

The bean-shaped **kidneys** are retroperitoneal, or posterior, to the abdominal contents. The spleen is a soft mass of lymphatic tissue on the posterolateral wall of the abdomen just under the diaphragm.

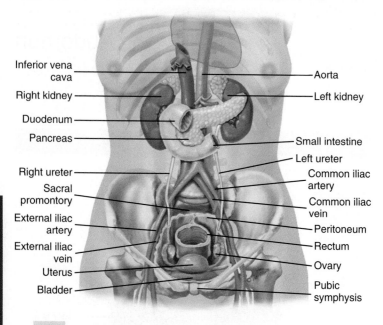

14.2 Relationship of aorta to deep abdominal viscera. (© Pat Thomas, 2006.)

SUBJECTIVE DATA

1. Change in appetite
2. Dysphagia (difficulty swallowing)
3. Food intolerance
4. Abdominal pain
5. Nausea/vomiting
6. Bowel habits
7. Rectal conditions
8. Past abdominal history (ulcer, gallbladder disease, hepatitis, appendicitis, colitis, hernia)
9. Medications (prescription, over-the-counter, including antacids)
10. Alcohol, drug, cigarette use
11. Nutritional assessment (24-hour recall)

OBJECTIVE DATA

PREPARATION

Turn on a strong overhead light and a secondary stand light. Expose the abdomen so it is fully visible. Drape the genitalia and female breasts.

The following measures enhance abdominal wall relaxation:

EQUIPMENT NEEDED

Stethoscope
Alcohol wipe (to clean endpiece)

- Have the person empty the bladder, saving a urine specimen if needed.
- Keep the room warm.
- Position the person supine with the head on a pillow, knees bent or on a pillow, and arms at the sides or across the chest.

- Keep the stethoscope endpiece warm, your hands warm, and your fingernails very short.
- Examine any painful areas last to avoid any muscle guarding.
- Use distraction: breathing exercises; emotive imagery; your low, soothing voice; and the person relating his or her abdominal history while you palpate.

Normal Range of Findings	Abnormal Findings

Inspect Contour, Symmetry, Umbilicus, Skin, Pulsation or Movement, and Demeanor

Contour. Stand on the person's right side and stoop to gaze across the abdomen. Determine the profile from the rib margin to the pubic bone, normally flat to rounded.

Protuberant abdomen, abdominal distention (see Table 14.1 on p. 180).
Scaphoid abdomen occurs with malnourishment.

Symmetry. Shine a light across the abdomen toward you or lengthwise across the person. The abdomen should be symmetric bilaterally. Note any localized bulging, visible mass, or asymmetry.

Bulges, masses.
Hernia—Protrusion of abdominal viscera through abnormal opening in muscle wall (see Table 22.4, p. 563, in Jarvis: *Physical Examination and Health Assessment,* 8th ed.).

Umbilicus. It is normally midline and inverted with no sign of discoloration, inflammation, or hernia. It becomes everted and pushed upward with pregnancy.

Everted with ascites or underlying mass.
Deeply sunken with obesity.
Enlarged and everted with umbilical hernia.

Skin. The surface is smooth and even, with homogeneous color.

Redness with localized inflammation; jaundice with hepatitis (shows best in natural daylight).
Skin glistening and taut with ascites.

Normally there are no lesions, although sometimes well-healed surgical scars are present. If a scar is present, draw its location in the person's record, indicating the length in centimeters.

Spider angiomas occur with portal hypertension or liver disease.
Lesions, rashes (see Chapter 5).

Pulsation or Movement. Pulsations from the aorta may show beneath the skin in the epigastric area, particularly in thin people with good muscle wall relaxation. Respiratory movement also shows in the abdomen, particularly in males.

Marked pulsation of the aorta with widened pulse pressure (e.g., hypertension, aortic insufficiency, thyrotoxicosis) and aortic aneurysm.
Marked visible peristalsis, together with a distended abdomen, indicates intestinal obstruction.

Normal Range of Findings	Abnormal Findings
Demeanor. A comfortable person is relaxed quietly on the examining table and has a benign facial expression and slow, even respirations.	Restlessness and constant turning to find comfort occur with the colicky pain of gastroenteritis or bowel obstruction. Absolute stillness, resisting any movement, is demonstrated with the pain of peritonitis. Knees flexed up, facial grimacing, and rapid, uneven respirations also indicate pain.

Auscultate Bowel Sounds and Vascular Sounds

Auscultation is done next because percussion and palpation can increase peristalsis, which would give a false interpretation of bowel sounds. Use the diaphragm endpiece and hold the stethoscope lightly against the skin. Begin in the right lower quadrant (RLQ) at the ileocecal valve area because bowel sounds normally are always present here.

Bowel Sounds. Note the character and frequency, normally high-pitched, gurgling, cascading sounds occurring irregularly, anywhere from 5 to 30 times per minute. Do not bother to count them. Judge if they are present, hypoactive, or hyperactive. You must listen for 5 minutes by your watch before deciding that bowel sounds are completely absent.

Two distinct patterns of abnormal bowel sounds may occur:

Hyperactive sounds are loud, high-pitched, rushing, tinkling sounds that signal increased motility. They occur with early mechanical bowel obstruction, gastroenteritis, brisk diarrhea, laxative use, and subsiding paralytic ileus.

Hypoactive or absent sounds follow abdominal surgery or occur with inflammation of the peritoneum or from late bowel obstruction (see Table 22.5, p. 564, in Jarvis: *Physical Examination and Health Assessment*, 8th ed.).

Vascular Sounds. Note the presence of any vascular sounds or *bruits*. Using firmer pressure, listen over the aorta, renal arteries, and iliac and femoral arteries, especially in people with hypertension (Fig. 14.3). Usually there is no such sound.

Note location, pitch, and timing of a vascular sound.

A systolic bruit is a pulsatile, blowing sound and occurs with stenosis, partial occlusion, or aneurysm of an artery.

Normal Range of Findings	Abnormal Findings

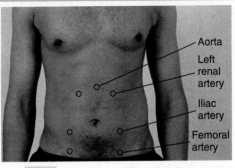

14.3 Sites to listen for vascular sounds.

Venous hum and peritoneal friction rub are rare (see Table 22.6, p. 565, in Jarvis: *Physical Examination and Health Assessment,* 8th ed.).

Percuss General Tympany, Liver Span, and Splenic Dullness

General Tympany. Percuss lightly in all four quadrants. Tympany should predominate because air in the intestines rises to the surface when the person is supine.

Liver Span. Traditionally, the upper and lower borders of the liver were identified by percussion to estimate liver span. This technique of measuring liver span underestimates the true liver size because clinicians place the upper border too low and/or the lower border too high (McGee, 2018). Percussion also yields highly variable results among examiners and frequently does not identify hepatomegaly even when present. Therefore, this examination technique is not recommended. Please see the information on palpation of the liver on p. 174 for further assessment.

Dullness occurs over a distended bladder, adipose tissue, fluid, or a mass.

Hyperresonance is present with gaseous distention.

Also, the upper liver border is overestimated if chronic obstructive lung disease is present, and both upper and lower edges are obscured if obesity or ascites is present.

Normal Range of Findings	Abnormal Findings

Splenic Dullness. By the same evidence, screening for splenomegaly through percussion of splenic dullness is omitted as detection through palpation is more reliable (McGee, 2018).

Palpate Surface and Deep Areas, Liver Edge, Spleen, and Kidneys

Light and Deep Palpation. Begin with **light palpation.** With the four fingers close together, depress the skin about 1 cm. Make a gentle rotary motion, lift the fingers (do not drag them), and move clockwise.

Muscle guarding.
Rigidity.
Large masses.
Tenderness.

As you circle the abdomen, discriminate between voluntary muscle guarding and involuntary rigidity. Voluntary **guarding** occurs when the person is cold, tense, or ticklish. It is bilateral, and the muscles relax slightly during exhalation. Use relaxation measures to try to eliminate this type of guarding or it will interfere with deep palpation. If rigidity persists, it probably is involuntary.

Involuntary **rigidity** is a constant, boardlike hardness of the muscles. It is a protective mechanism accompanying acute inflammation of the peritoneum. It may be unilateral, and the same area usually becomes painful when the person increases intra-abdominal pressure by attempting a sit-up.

Now perform **deep palpation,** pushing down about 5 to 8 cm (2 to 3 inches). Moving clockwise, explore the entire abdomen.

To overcome the resistance of a very large or obese abdomen, use a bimanual technique. Place your hands on top of one another. The top hand pushes; the bottom hand is relaxed and can concentrate on the sense of palpation. With either technique note the location, size, consistency, and mobility of any palpable organs and the presence of any abnormal enlargement, tenderness, or masses. Remember that some structures are normally palpable, as illustrated in Fig. 14.4.

Normal Range of Findings	Abnormal Findings

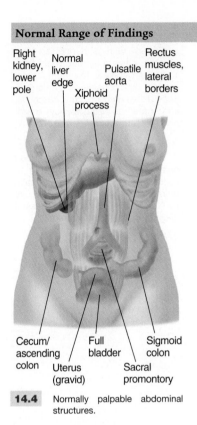

Right kidney, lower pole

Normal liver edge

Xiphoid process

Pulsatile aorta

Rectus muscles, lateral borders

Cecum/ ascending colon

Uterus (gravid)

Full bladder

Sacral promontory

Sigmoid colon

14.4 Normally palpable abdominal structures.

Normally there is mild tenderness when palpating the sigmoid colon. Any other tenderness should be investigated.

If you identify a mass, first distinguish it from a normally palpable structure or an enlarged organ. Then note its:
1. Location
2. Size
3. Shape
4. Consistency (soft, firm, hard)
5. Surface (smooth, nodular)
6. Mobility (including movement with respirations)
7. Pulsatility
8. Tenderness

Tenderness occurs with local inflammation, with inflammation of the peritoneum or underlying organ, and with an enlarged organ whose capsule is stretched.

Normal Range of Findings	Abnormal Findings

Liver. Place your left hand under the person's back, parallel to the 11th and 12th ribs, and lift up to support the abdominal contents. Place your right hand on the right upper quadrant (RUQ), with fingers parallel to the midline (Fig. 14.5). Push deeply down and under the right costal margin. Ask the person to take a deep breath. It is normal to feel the edge of the liver bump your fingertips as the diaphragm pushes it down during inhalation. It feels like a firm, regular ridge. The liver is often not palpable, and you may feel nothing firm.

Except with a depressed diaphragm, a liver palpated more than 1 to 2 cm below the right costal margin is considered enlarged. Record the number of cm it descends, and note its consistency (hard, nodular) and any tenderness.

The liver edge is often palpated below the right costal margin in people with chronic obstructive pulmonary disease (COPD) because their distended lungs and depressed diaphragm push the liver lower.

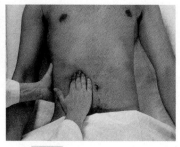

14.5 Palpating the liver.

Spleen. Normally the spleen is not palpable and must be enlarged 3 times its normal size to be felt. Reach your left hand over the abdomen and behind the left side at the 11th and 12th ribs. Lift up for support. Place your right hand obliquely on the LUQ with the fingers pointing toward the left axilla and just inferior to the rib margin. Push your hand deeply down and under the left costal margin, and ask the person to take a deep breath. You should feel nothing firm. When enlarged, the spleen slides out and bumps your fingertips.

The spleen enlarges with mononucleosis and trauma (see Table 22.7, p. 566, in Jarvis: *Physical Examination and Health Assessment,* 8th ed.). Refer the person with an enlarged spleen; do not continue to palpate. An enlarged spleen is friable and can rupture easily with overpalpation.

Describe the number of cm it extends below the left costal margin.

Normal Range of Findings	Abnormal Findings

Kidneys. Search for the right kidney by placing your hands together in a "duckbill" position at the person's right flank. Press your two hands firmly and ask the person to take a deep breath. With most people, you feel no change. Occasionally you may feel the lower pole of the right kidney as a round, smooth mass slide between your fingers. Either condition is normal.

The left kidney sits 1 cm higher than the right kidney and normally is not palpable.

Aorta. Using your opposing thumb and fingers, palpate the aortic pulsation in the upper abdomen slightly to the left of midline. It is normally 2.5 to 4 cm wide in adults and pulsates in an anterior direction.

Costovertebral Angle Tenderness. Place one hand over the 12th rib at the costovertebral angle on the back. Thump that hand with the ulnar edge of your other fist. The person normally feels a thud but no pain.

Special Procedures

Rebound Tenderness. Choose a site remote from the painful area. Hold your hand 90 degrees or perpendicular to the abdomen. Push down slowly and deeply; then lift up *quickly*. This makes structures that are indented by palpation rebound suddenly. A normal, or negative, response is absence of pain on release of pressure. Perform this test at the end of the examination because it can cause severe pain and muscle rigidity.

Fluid Wave for Ascites. Place the ulnar edge of another examiner's hand or the patient's own hand firmly on the abdomen midline (Fig. 14.6). Place your left hand on the person's right flank. With your right hand

Enlarged kidney.
Kidney mass.

Widened aorta with aneurysm.
Prominent lateral pulsation with aortic aneurysm (see Table 22.6, p. 567, in Jarvis: *Physical Examination and Health Assessment*, 8th ed.).

Sharp pain occurs with inflammation of the kidney or paranephric area.

Pain on release of pressure confirms rebound tenderness, which is a reliable sign of peritoneal inflammation.

Cough tenderness localized to a specific spot also signals peritoneal irritation.

Normal Range of Findings	Abnormal Findings

reach across the abdomen and give the left flank a firm strike. If ascites is present, the blow will generate a fluid wave through the abdomen and you will feel a distinct tap on your left hand. If the abdomen is distended from gas or adipose tissue, you will feel no change.

Ascites occurs with heart failure, portal hypertension, cirrhosis, hepatitis, pancreatitis, and cancer.

A positive fluid wave test occurs with large amounts of ascitic fluid.

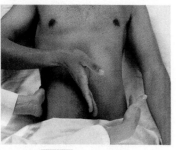

14.6 Fluid wave.

◆ DEVELOPMENTAL COMPETENCE

The Infant

The contour of the abdomen is protuberant because of the immature abdominal musculature. The skin contains a fine, superficial venous pattern. This may be visible in children until puberty.

Scaphoid shape occurs with dehydration or malnutrition.
Dilated veins.

The abdomen shows respiratory movement. The only other abdominal movement is occasional peristalsis, which may be visible because of the thin musculature.

Marked peristalsis occurs with pyloric stenosis.

Auscultation yields only bowel sounds, the metallic tinkling of peristalsis. There should be no vascular sounds.

Bruit indicates stenosis or obstruction.

Aid palpation by flexing the baby's knees with one hand while palpating with the other (Fig. 14.7).

Normal Range of Findings	Abnormal Findings

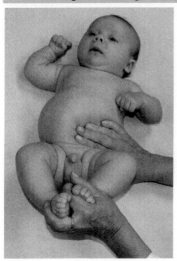

14.7

The liver fills the RUQ. It is normal to feel the liver edge at the right costal margin or 1 to 2 cm below. Normally you may palpate the spleen tip and both kidneys and the bladder. Also easily palpated are the cecum in the RLQ and the sigmoid colon, which feels like a sausage in the left inguinal area.

The Child

In children younger than age 4 years, the abdomen looks protuberant when the child is both supine and standing. After age 4 years the pot belly remains when standing because of lumbar lordosis, but the abdomen looks flat when supine. Normal movement on the abdomen includes respirations, which remain abdominal until 7 years of age.

A scaphoid abdomen is associated with dehydration or malnutrition.

In children younger than 7 years of age the absence of abdominal respirations occurs with inflammation of the peritoneum.

Normal Range of Findings	Abnormal Findings

The Aging Adult

On inspection you may note increased deposits of subcutaneous fat on the abdomen and hips as it is redistributed away from the extremities. The abdominal musculature is thinner and has less tone than that of the younger adult; therefore in the absence of obesity you may note peristalsis.

Because of the thinner, softer abdominal wall, the organs may be easier to palpate (in the absence of obesity). The liver is easier to palpate. Normally you feel the liver edge at or just below the costal margin. With distended lungs and a depressed diaphragm, the liver is palpated lower, descending 1 to 2 cm below the costal margin with inhalation. The kidneys are easier to palpate.

Abdominal rigidity with acute abdominal conditions is less common in older adults.

With an acute abdomen an older adult often complains of less pain than would a younger person.

HEALTH PROMOTION AND PATIENT TEACHING

Hepatitis B and Hepatitis C

I would like to have a conversation about your potential risks for viral hepatitis, which is a liver infection. There are three major types of hepatitis: A, B, and C. Hepatitis B and C are spread through blood and body fluids, for example by sharing contaminated needles or by sexual contact. Both hepatitis B and C can cause a brief period of illness, then either be cleared from the body entirely or go on to cause a long-term, or chronic, infection. Chronic infection is especially common with hepatitis C. If the hepatitis becomes a chronic infection, it can eventually cause the liver to fail by causing liver scarring (fibrosis and cirrhosis). Chronic hepatitis also increases your risk for liver cancer.

High-risk individuals should be screened for hepatitis B and C through blood testing and referred to appropriate providers for treatment if testing is positive. Primary prevention includes risk factor modification and vaccination against hepatitis B for appropriate individuals.

Summary Checklist: Abdomen

1. **Inspection:**
   Contour
   Symmetry
   Skin
   Pulsation or movement
   Demeanor
2. **Auscultation:**
   Bowel sounds
   Vascular sounds
3. **Percussion:**
   All four quadrants
4. **Palpation:**
   Light palpation in all four quadrants
   Deep palpation in all four quadrants
   Liver, spleen, kidneys

DOCUMENTATION

Sample Charting

SUBJECTIVE

States appetite is good with no recent change, no dysphagia, no food intolerance, no pain, no nausea/vomiting. Has one formed BM/day. Takes OTC multivitamins, no other prescribed or over-the-counter medication. No history of abdominal disease, injury, or surgery. Diet recall of past 24 hours listed at end of history.

OBJECTIVE

Inspection: Abdomen flat, symmetric, with no apparent masses. Skin smooth with no striae, scars, or lesions.
Auscultation: Bowel sounds present, no bruits.
Percussion: Tympany predominates in all 4 quadrants.
Palpation: Abdomen soft, no organomegaly, no masses, no tenderness.

ASSESSMENT

Healthy abdomen, bowel sounds present

ABNORMAL FINDINGS

TABLE 14.1	Abdominal Distention

Obesity

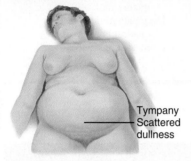

Tympany
Scattered
dullness

Air or Gas

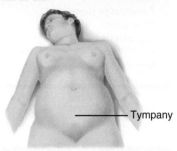

— Tympany

Inspection. Uniformly rounded. Umbilicus sunken (it adheres to peritoneum, and layers of fat are superficial to it).
Auscultation. Normal bowel sounds.
Percussion. Tympany. Scattered dullness over adipose tissue.
Palpation. Normal. May be hard to feel through thick abdominal wall.

Inspection. Single round curve.
Auscultation. Depends on cause of gas (e.g., decreased or absent bowel sounds with ileus); hyperactive with early intestinal obstruction.
Percussion. Tympany over large area.
Palpation. May have muscle spasm of abdominal wall.

Ascites

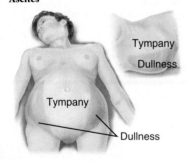

Tympany

Dullness

Tympany

Dullness

◀ **Inspection.** Single curve. Everted umbilicus. Bulging flanks when supine. Taut, glistening skin due to recent weight gain; increase in abdominal girth.
Auscultation. Normal bowel sounds over intestines. Diminished over ascitic fluid.
Percussion. Tympany at top where intestines float. Dull over fluid. Produces fluid wave and shifting dullness.
Palpation. Taut skin and increased intra-abdominal pressure limit palpation.

Continued

TABLE 14.1 Abdominal Distention—cont'd

Ovarian Cyst (Large)

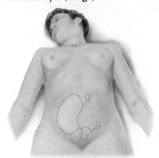

Inspection. Curve in lower half of abdomen, midline. Everted umbilicus.

Auscultation. Normal bowel sounds over upper abdomen where intestines pushed superiorly.

Percussion. Top dull over fluid. Intestines pushed superiorly. Large cyst produces fluid wave and shifting dullness.

Palpation. Transmits aortic pulsation, whereas ascites does not.

Pregnancy

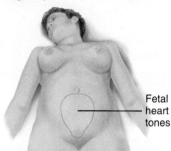

Fetal heart tones

Inspection. Single curve. Umbilicus protruding. Breasts engorged.

Auscultation. Fetal heart tones. Bowel sounds diminished.

Percussion. Tympany over intestines. Dull over enlarging uterus.

Palpation. Uterine fundus. Fetal parts. Fetal movements.

Feces

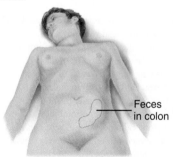

Feces in colon

Inspection. Localized distention.

Auscultation. Normal bowel sounds.

Percussion. Tympany predominates. Scattered dullness over fecal mass.

Palpation. Plastic or ropelike mass with feces in intestines.

Tumor

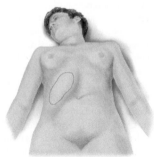

Inspection. Localized distention.

Auscultation. Normal bowel sounds.

Percussion. Dull over mass if reaches up to skin surface.

Palpation. Define borders. Distinguish from enlarged organ or normally palpable structure.

TABLE 14.2   Common Sites of Referred Abdominal Pain

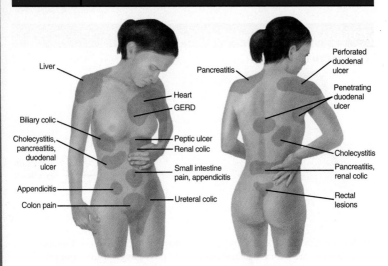

Abdominal pain may be referred to a site where the organ was located in fetal development. The following are examples:

Liver. Hepatitis may have mild-to-moderate, dull pain in right upper quadrant (RUQ) or epigastrium, along with anorexia, nausea, malaise, low-grade fever.

Esophagus. Gastroesophageal reflux disease (GERD) is a complex of symptoms of esophagitis, including burning pain in midepigastrium or behind lower sternum that radiates upward (i.e., heartburn). Occurs 30 to 60 minutes after eating; aggravated by lying down or bending over.

Gallbladder. Cholecystitis is biliary colic, i.e., sudden pain in right upper quadrant that may radiate to right or left scapula and that builds over time, lasting 2 to 4 hours, after ingestion of fatty foods, alcohol, or caffeine. Associated with nausea and vomiting and with positive Murphy sign or sudden stop in inspiration with RUQ palpation.

Pancreas. Pancreatitis has acute, boring midepigastric pain radiating to the back and sometimes to the left scapula or flank, severe nausea and vomiting.

Duodenum. Duodenal ulcer typically has dull, aching, gnawing pain; does not radiate, may be relieved by food; and may awaken the person from sleep.

Stomach. Gastric ulcer pain is dull, aching, gnawing epigastric pain, usually brought on by food; radiates to back or substernal area. Pain of perforated ulcer is burning epigastric pain of sudden onset that refers to one or both shoulders.

Appendix. Appendicitis typically starts as dull, diffuse pain in periumbilical region that later shifts to severe, sharp, persistent pain and tenderness localized in RLQ (McBurney point). Pain is aggravated by movement, coughing, deep breathing; associated with anorexia, then nausea and vomiting, fever.

Kidney. Kidney stones prompt a sudden onset of severe, colicky flank or lower abdominal pain.

Small intestine. Gastroenteritis has diffuse, generalized abdominal pain with nausea, diarrhea.

Colon. Large bowel obstruction has moderate, colicky pain of gradual onset in lower abdomen, bloating. Irritable bowel syndrome (IBS) has sharp or burning, cramping pain over a wide area; does not radiate. Brought on by meals, relieved by bowel movement.

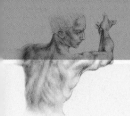

CHAPTER 15

Musculoskeletal System

ANATOMY

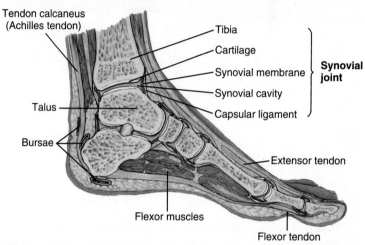

Tendon calcaneus (Achilles tendon)

Tibia

Cartilage

Synovial membrane

Synovial cavity

Capsular ligament

Synovial joint

Talus

Bursae

Extensor tendon

Flexor muscles

Flexor tendon

15.1 Components of a synovial joint.

The musculoskeletal system consists of the bones, joints, and muscles.

A **joint** (or articulation) is the place of union of two or more bones. Joints are the functional units of the musculoskeletal system because they permit the mobility needed for activities of daily living (ADL).

Synovial joints are freely movable because their bones are separated from one another and enclosed in a joint cavity (Fig. 15.1). This cavity is filled with a lubricant called *synovial fluid*.

In synovial joints a layer of resilient **cartilage** covers the surface of opposing bones. The cartilage cushions the bones and gives a smooth surface to facilitate movement. The joint is surrounded by a fibrous capsule and is supported by ligaments. **Ligaments** are fibrous bands running directly from one bone to another that strengthen the joint and help prevent movement in undesirable directions. A **bursa** is an enclosed sac filled with viscous synovial fluid, much like a joint. Bursae are located in areas of potential friction (e.g., subacromial bursa of the shoulder, prepatellar bursa of the knee) and help muscles and tendons glide smoothly over bone.

Skeletal **muscle** is attached to bone by a **tendon**—a strong fibrous cord.

183

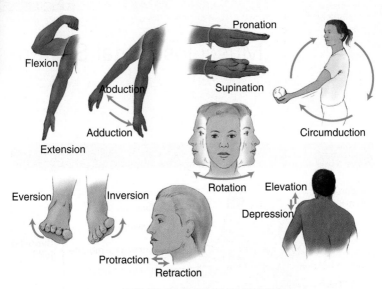

Pronation

Supination

Flexion

Abduction

Adduction

Extension

Circumduction

Eversion   Inversion

Rotation   Elevation

Depression

Protraction

Retraction

SKELETAL MUSCLE MOVEMENTS

15.2

(© Pat Thomas, 2006.)

Skeletal muscles produce the following movements (Fig. 15.2):

1. Flexion—bending a limb at a joint
2. Extension—straightening a limb at a joint
3. Abduction—moving a limb away from the midline of the body
4. Adduction—moving a limb toward the midline of the body
5. Pronation—turning the forearm so the palm is down
6. Supination—turning the forearm so the palm is up
7. Circumduction—moving the arm in a circle around the shoulder
8. Inversion—moving the sole of the foot inward at the ankle
9. Eversion—moving the sole of the foot outward at the ankle
10. Rotation—moving the head around a central axis
11. Protraction—moving a body part forward and parallel to the ground
12. Retraction—moving a body part backward and parallel to the ground
13. Elevation—raising a body part
14. Depression—lowering a body part

CULTURE AND GENETICS

Substantial racial/ethnic differences exist in bone mineral density (BMD) among women in the United States and globally. A higher BMD value means a denser bone; a low BMD value is a strong and consistent predictor of hip and vertebral fracture among postmenopausal women. Evidence comparing BMD in older women in four countries showed that, compared with U.S. Caucasian women, the BMD hip site measurements were 21% to 31% higher in Afro-Caribbean women and 13% to 23% higher in African-American women, similar in Hong Kong Chinese women, and higher in South Korean women (Nam, et al., 2013). The higher BMD values confer a lower fracture risk among women of African heritage.

In the spine women of all races gained BMD up to age 30 to 33 years (Berenson, Rahman, & Wilkinson, 2009). But at the femoral neck in the hip joint, BMD peaked earlier among white women (≤16 years) than among African Americans (21 years) and Hispanics (20 years). An earlier peak BMD followed by a more rapid decline is a trend that may explain the increased fracture risk for white women later in life. These data, plus physical activity data, suggest that weight-bearing physical activity (such as fast walking) is imperative during teen, early adult, and middle adult years to slow the process of decline in BMD.

SUBJECTIVE DATA

1. Joints
   Pain
   Stiffness
   Swelling, heat
   Limitation of movement
2. Muscles
   Pain (cramps)
   Weakness
3. Bones
   Pain
   Deformity
   Trauma (fractures, sprains, dislocations)
4. Functional assessment (ADL)
   Any self-care deficit in bathing, toileting, dressing, grooming, eating, communicating, mobility
   Use of mobility aids
5. Patient-centered care
   Occupational hazards
   Heavy lifting
   Repetitive motion to joints
   Nature of exercise program
   Recent weight gain

OBJECTIVE DATA

PREPARATION

A **screening musculoskeletal** examination suffices for most people:

- Inspection and palpation of joints integrated with each body region
- Observation of range of motion (ROM) as person proceeds through motions necessary for an examination
- Age-specific screening measures, e.g., scoliosis screening for adolescents when indicated

A **complete musculoskeletal** examination, as described in this chapter, is appropriate for people with articular disease, a history of musculoskeletal symptoms, or any problems with ADL.

EQUIPMENT NEEDED

Tape measure
Skin-marking pen

Normal Range of Findings	Abnormal Findings

Order of the Examination

Inspection

Compare corresponding paired joints. Inspect for symmetry of structure and function and normal parameters for that joint.

Note the *size* and *contour* of the joint. Inspect the skin and tissues over the joints for color, swelling, and masses or deformity.

Presence of swelling is significant and signals joint irritation.

Palpation

Palpate each joint, including its skin, for temperature, its muscles, bony articulations, and area of joint capsule. Notice any heat, tenderness, swelling, and masses. Joints are normally not tender to palpation.

Heat, tenderness, and swelling signal inflammation.
Palpable fluid.

Range of Motion

Ask for **active** ROM while stabilizing the body area proximal to that being moved. Familiarize yourself with the type of each joint and its normal ROM so you can recognize limitations.

Joint motion normally causes no tenderness, pain, or crepitation. Do not confuse crepitation with the normal, discrete "crack" heard as a tendon or ligament slips over bone during motion such as knee bends.

If you see a limitation, gently attempt **passive** motion. Anchor the joint with one hand while your other hand slowly moves it to its limit. The normal ranges of active and passive motion should be the same.

Crepitation is an audible and palpable crunching or grating that accompanies movement. It occurs when the articular surfaces in the joints are roughened, as with rheumatoid arthritis (see Table 15.1 on p. 201).

Muscle Testing

Test the strength of the prime-mover muscle groups for each joint. Repeat the motions that you elicited for active ROM. Ask the person to flex and hold as you apply opposing force. Muscle strength should be equal bilaterally and should fully resist your opposing force. (NOTE: Muscle status and joint status are interdependent and should be interpreted together. Chapter 16 discusses the examination of muscles for size and development, tone, and presence of tenderness.)

Strength varies widely among people. Use a grading system from no voluntary movement to full strength, as shown in Table 15.2 on p. 202.

Normal Range of Findings	Abnormal Findings

Cervical Spine

Inspect the alignment of head and neck. The spine should be straight and the head erect. Palpate the spinous processes and the sternomastoid, trapezius, and paravertebral muscles. They should feel firm, with no muscle spasm or tenderness.

Head tilted to one side.

Asymmetry of muscles.
Tenderness (musle spasm, postural disorders or arthritis).
Hard muscles with muscle spasm.

Ask the person to follow these motions[a]:

Instructions to Person	Motion and Expected Range
• Touch chin to chest.	Flexion of 45 degrees.
• Lift chin toward the ceiling.	Hyperextension of 55 degrees.
• Touch each ear toward the corresponding shoulder. Do not lift the shoulder.	Lateral bending of 40 degrees.
• Turn chin toward each shoulder.	Rotation of 70 degrees.

Limited ROM (arthritis).
Pain with movement.

Repeat the motions while applying opposing force. The person can normally maintain flexion against your full resistance. This also tests the integrity of cranial nerve XI.

The person cannot hold flexion.

Upper Extremity

Shoulder

Inspect and compare both shoulders posteriorly and anteriorly. Check the size and contour of the joint and compare shoulders for equality of bony landmarks. Normally there is no redness, muscular atrophy, deformity, or swelling.

Redness.
Inequality of bony landmarks.
Atrophy shows as lack of fullness (see Table 23.2, p. 613, in Jarvis: *Physical Examination and Health Assessment,* 8th ed.).

While standing in front of the person, **palpate** both shoulders, noting any muscular spasm or atrophy, swelling, heat, or tenderness.

Swelling.
Hard muscles with muscle spasm.

[a]DO NOT ATTEMPT IF YOU SUSPECT NECK TRAUMA.

Normal Range of Findings	Abnormal Findings

Test **ROM** by asking the person to perform four motions. Cup one hand over the shoulder during ROM to note any crepitation; normally there is none.

Tenderness or pain.

Instructions to Person	Motion and Expected Range
1. With arms at sides and elbows extended, move both arms forward and up in wide vertical arcs. Then move them back.	Forward flexion of 180 degrees. Hyperextension up to 50 degrees.
2. Rotate arms internally behind back; place back of hands as high as possible toward the scapulae.	Internal rotation of 90 degrees.
3. With arms at sides and elbows extended, raise both arms in wide arcs in the coronal plane. Touch palms together above head.	Abduction of 180 degrees. Adduction of 50 degrees.
4. Touch both hands behind the head, with elbows flexed and rotated posteriorly.	External rotation of 90 degrees.

Limited ROM.
Asymmetry.
Pain with motion.
Crepitus with motion.

Test the **strength** of the shoulder muscles by asking the person to shrug his or her shoulders, flex forward and up, and abduct against your resistance. The shoulder shrug also tests the integrity of cranial nerve XI, the spinal accessory.

Elbow

Inspect the size and contour of the elbow in both flexed and extended positions. Look for any deformity, redness, or swelling.

Swelling and redness (see Table 23.3, p. 614, in Jarvis: *Physical Examination and Health Assessment*, 8th ed.).

Normal Range of Findings	Abnormal Findings

Test **ROM** by asking the person to:

Instructions to Person	Motion and Expected Range
• Bend and straighten the elbow.	Flexion of 150 to 160 degrees, extension at 0. Some normal people lack 5 to 10 degrees of full extension, and others have 5 to 10 degrees of hyperextension.
• Hold the hand midway; then touch front and back sides of hand to table.	Movement of 90 degrees in pronation and supination.

While testing **muscle strength**, stabilize the person's arm with one hand (Fig. 15.3). Have the person flex the elbow against your resistance, applied just proximal to the wrist. Then ask him or her to extend the elbow against your resistance.

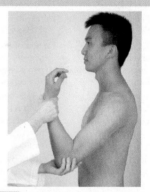

15.3 Stabilize the joint while testing muscle strength.

Wrist and Hand

Inspect the hands and wrists on the dorsal and palmar sides, noting position, contour, and shape. The normal functional position of the hand shows the wrist in slight extension. This way the fingers can flex efficiently, and the thumb can oppose them for grip and manipulation. The fingers lie straight in the same axis as the forearm. There is normally no swelling or redness, deformity, or nodules.

Subluxation of wrist.

Ulnar deviation—Fingers list to ulnar side.

Ankylosing—Wrist in extreme flexion.

Dupuytren contracture—Flexion contracture of fingers.

Swan-neck or boutonnière deformity in fingers.

Hard nodules on fingers (see Table 23.4, p. 616, in Jarvis: *Physical Examination and Health Assessment*, 8th ed.).

Normal Range of Findings	Abnormal Findings

The skin looks smooth, with knuckle wrinkles present and no swelling or lesions. Muscles are full, with the palm showing a rounded mound proximal to the thumb (the *thenar eminence*) and a smaller rounded mound proximal to the little finger.

Atrophy of thenar eminence occurs with carpal tunnel syndrome as a result of compression of the median nerve.

Palpate each joint in the wrist and hands. Facing the person, support the hand with your fingers under it. Use gentle but firm pressure. Normally the joint surfaces feel smooth, with no swelling, bogginess, nodules, or tenderness.

Ganglion in wrist—localized hard nodule.
Synovial swelling on dorsum.
Generalized swelling.
Tenderness.

Test **ROM** with this procedure:

Instructions to Person	Motion and Expected Range
• Bend hand up at the wrist.	Hyperextension of 70 degrees.
• Bend hand down at the wrist.	Palmar flexion of 90 degrees.
• Bend fingers up and down at metacarpophalangeal joints.	Flexion of 90 degrees. Hyperextension of 30 degrees.
• With palms flat on table, turn them outward and in.	Ulnar deviation of 50 to 60 degrees; radial deviation of 20 degrees.
• Spread fingers apart; make a fist.	Abduction of 20 degrees; fist tight. The responses should be equal bilaterally.
• Touch thumb to each finger and to base of little finger.	The person is able to perform, and the responses are equal bilaterally.

Loss of ROM here is the most common and most significant type of function loss of the wrist.
Limited motion.
Pain on movement.

Lower Extremity

Hip

Wait to **inspect** the hip joint together with the spine a bit later in the examination as the person stands. At that time note symmetric levels of iliac

Normal Range of Findings	Abnormal Findings

crests, gluteal folds, and equally sized buttocks. A smooth, even gait reflects equal leg lengths and functional hip motion.

Help the person into a supine position and **palpate** the hip joints. The joints should feel stable and symmetric, with no tenderness or crepitation.

Pain with palpation.

Crepitation.

Assess **ROM** by asking the person to:

Instructions to Person	Motion and Expected Range	
• Raise each leg with knee extended.	Hip flexion of 90 degrees.	Limited motion. Pain with motion.
• Bend each knee up to the chest while keeping the other leg straight.	Hip flexion of 120 degrees. The opposite thigh should remain on the table.	Flexion flattens the lumbar spine; if this reveals a flexion deformity in the opposite hip, it is abnormal.
• Flex knee and hip to 90 degrees. Stabilize by holding the thigh with one hand and the ankle with the other hand. Swing foot outward. Swing foot inward. (Foot and thigh move in opposing directions.)	Internal rotation of 40 degrees. External rotation of 45 degrees.	Limited internal rotation of hip is an early and reliable sign of hip disease.
• Swing leg laterally, then medially, with knee straight. Stabilize pelvis by pushing down on the opposite anterior superior iliac spine.	Abduction of 40 to 45 degrees; adduction of 20 to 30 degrees.	Limitation of abduction of the hip while supine is the most common motion dysfunction found in hip disease.
• When standing (later in examination), swing straight leg back behind body. Stabilize pelvis to eliminate exaggerated lumbar lordosis.	Hyperextension of 15 degrees when stabilized.	

Normal Range of Findings	Abnormal Findings

Knee

The skin normally looks smooth, with even coloring and free of lesions.

Calluses.
Shiny and atrophic skin.
Inflammation.
Lesions (e.g., psoriasis).

Inspect lower leg alignment. The lower leg should extend in the same axis as the thigh.

Angulation deformity.
Flexion contracture.

Inspect the knee's shape and contour. Normally there are distinct concavities, or hollows, on either side of the patella. Check them for any sign of fullness or swelling. Note other locations such as the prepatellar bursa and the suprapatellar pouch for any abnormal swelling.

Hollows disappear and then may bulge with synovial thickening or effusion (see Table 23.5, p. 618, in Jarvis: *Physical Examination and Health Assessment,* 8th ed.).

Check quadriceps muscle in the anterior thigh for any atrophy. Because it is the prime mover of knee extension, this muscle is important for joint stability during weight bearing.

Atrophy occurs with disuse or chronic disorders. It first appears in the medial part of the muscle, although it is difficult to note because the vastus medialis is relatively small.

Check **ROM** by asking the person to:

Instructions to Person	Motion and Expected Range	
• Bend each knee.	Flexion of 130 to 150 degrees.	Limited ROM.
• Extend each knee.	A straight line of 0 degrees in some people; a hyperextension of 15 degrees in others.	Contracture. Pain with motion.
• Check knee ROM during ambulation.		Limp. Sudden locking—The person is unable to extend the knee fully. This usually occurs with a painful and audible "pop" or "click." Sudden buckling, or "giving way," occurs with ligament injury, which causes weakness and instability.

Check muscle **strength** by asking the person to maintain knee flexion while you oppose by trying to pull the leg forward. Muscle extension is demonstrated by the person's success in rising from a seated position in a low chair or by rising from a squat without using the hands for support.

Normal Range of Findings	Abnormal Findings

Ankle and Foot

Inspect and compare both feet, noting position of feet and toes, contour of joints, and skin characteristics. The foot should align with the long axis of the lower leg.

The toes point straight forward and lie flat. The ankles (malleoli) are smooth, bony prominences. The skin is normally smooth, with even coloring and no lesions. Note the locations of any calluses or bursal reactions because they reveal areas of abnormal friction. Examining well-worn shoes helps assess areas of wear and accommodation.

Hallux valgus (toe pointing outward from midline) and bunion.
Hammertoes.
Swelling or inflammation.

Calluses. Bunions.
Ulcers.
(See Table 23.6, p. 619, in Jarvis: *Physical Examination and Health Assessment,* 8th ed.).

Test **ROM** by asking the person to:

Instructions to Person	Motion and Expected Range
• Point toes toward the floor.	Plantar flexion of 45 degrees.
• Point toes toward your nose.	Dorsiflexion of 20 degrees.
• Turn soles of feet out and then in. (Stabilize ankle with one hand and hold heel with the other to test the subtalar joint.)	Eversion of 20 degrees. Inversion of 30 degrees.
• Flex and straighten toes.	

Limited ROM.
Pain with motion.

Assess muscle **strength** by asking the person to maintain dorsiflexion and plantar flexion against your resistance.

Unable to hold flexion.

Spine

The person should be standing, draped in a gown open at the back. Place yourself far enough back so you can see the entire back. Note if the spine is straight by following an imaginary vertical line from the head through the spinous processes and down through the gluteal cleft and by noting equal horizontal positions for the shoulders,

Normal Range of Findings	Abnormal Findings

scapulae, iliac crests, and gluteal folds and equal spaces between arm and lateral thorax on the two sides (Fig. 15-4, *A*). The person's knees and feet should be aligned with the trunk and should be pointing forward.

A difference in shoulder elevation and in level of scapulae and iliac crests occurs with scoliosis.

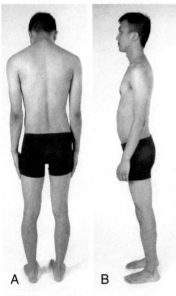

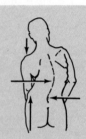

Scoliosis ▲
A lateral S-shaped curvature of the thoracic and lumbar spine, usually with involved vertebrae rotation. Note rib hump on forward flexion. When standing, note unequal shoulder and scapular height, obvious curvature, unequal elbow level, unequal hip levels, and rib interspaces flared on convex side. More prevalent in adolescence, especially in girls.

15.4   **A,** Straight spine. **B,** Normal curvature seen from side.

The vertebral column has four curves (a double-S shape). From the side note the normal convex thoracic curve and concave lumbar curve (see Fig. 15-4, *B*). The cervical and lumbar curves are concave (inward), and the thoracic and sacrococcygeal curves are convex. The balanced or compensatory nature of these curves, together with the resilient intervertebral disks, allows the spine to absorb a great deal of shock.

An enhanced thoracic curve, or **kyphosis**, is common in older adults. A pronounced lumbar curve, or **lordosis**, is common in obese people.

Lateral tilting and forward bending occur with a herniated nucleus pulposus from pressure on the local spinal nerve root. ▼

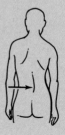

Normal Range of Findings	Abnormal Findings

Check **ROM** of the spine by asking the person to bend forward and touch the toes. Look for flexion of 75 to 90 degrees and smoothness and symmetry of movement. Note that the concave lumbar curve should disappear with this motion and the back should have a single, convex, C-shaped curve.

Stabilize the pelvis with your hands. Check **ROM** by asking the person to:

Instructions to Person	Motion and Expected Range	
• Bend sideways.	Lateral bending of 35 degrees.	Limited ROM.
• Bend backward.	Hyperextension of 30 degrees.	Pain with motion.
• Twist shoulders to one side and then the other.	Rotation of 30 degrees bilaterally.	

 DEVELOPMENTAL COMPETENCE

Infants

Lift the infant and examine the back. Note the normal, single, C-curve of the newborn's spine (Fig. 15.5). By 2 months of age the infant can lift the head while prone. This builds the concave cervical spinal curve and indicates normal forearm strength.

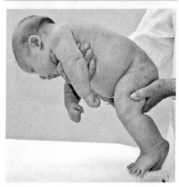

15.5 Normal spinal curvature in newborn.

Observe ROM through spontaneous movement of extremities.

Test muscle strength by lifting the infant with your hands under the baby's axillae. A baby with normal muscle strength wedges securely between your hands.

A baby who starts to slip between your hands shows weakness of the shoulder muscles.

Normal Range of Findings	Abnormal Findings

Preschool and School-Age Children

You can observe the muscles and joints during spontaneous play before a table-top examination. Most young children enjoy showing off their physical accomplishments. For specific motions coax the toddler: "Show me how you can walk to Mom," or, "Climb the stepstool." Ask the preschooler to hop on one foot or jump (Fig. 15.6).

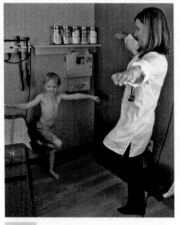

15.6

While the child is standing, note the posture. From behind you should note a "plumb line" from the back of the head, along the spine, to the middle of the sacrum. Shoulders are level within 1 cm, and scapulae are symmetric. From the side lordosis is common throughout childhood, appearing more pronounced in children with a protuberant abdomen.

Check the child's gait while walking away from and returning to you. Let the child wear socks because a cold tile floor will distort the usual gait.

Lordosis is marked with muscular dystrophy and rickets.

Normal Range of Findings	Abnormal Findings

From 1 to 2 years of age expect a broad-based gait, with arms out for balance. Weight-bearing falls on the inside of the foot. From 3 years of age the base narrows, and the arms are closer to the sides. Inspect the shoes for spots of greatest wear to aid your judgment of the gait. Normally the shoes wear more on the outside of the heel and the inside of the toe.

Limp; usually caused by trauma, fatigue, or hip disease.

Adolescents

Proceed with the musculoskeletal examination that you provide for the adult, except pay special note to spinal posture. Kyphosis is common during adolescence because of chronic poor posture.

Screen for **scoliosis** only when indicated (incidental finding or parental concern). Seat yourself behind the standing child and ask him or her to bend forward to touch the toes. Expect a straight vertical spine while standing and also while bending forward. Posterior ribs should be symmetric, with equal elevation of shoulders, scapulae, and iliac crests.

Scoliosis is exhibited as ribs hump up on one side as child bends forward and with unequal shoulder or hip landmark elevation (see p. 194).

Be aware of the risk of sports-related injuries with the adolescent because sports participation and competition reach a height with this age-group.

The Pregnant Woman

Proceed through the examination described in the adult section. Expected postural changes in pregnancy include progressive lordosis and, toward the third trimester, anterior cervical flexion, kyphosis, and slumped shoulders (Fig. 15-7, *A* and *B*). When the pregnancy is at term, the protuberant abdomen and relaxed mobility in the joints create the characteristic "waddling" gait.

Normal Range of Findings	Abnormal Findings

15.7 Postural changes in pregnancy.

The Aging Adult

Postural changes include a decrease in height, more apparent in the 70s and 80s (Fig. 15.8). "Lengthening of the arm-trunk axis" describes this shortening of the trunk with comparatively long extremities. **Kyphosis** is common, with a backward head tilt to compensate and maintain the level of vision. This creates the outline of a figure 3 when you view this older adult from the left side. Slight flexion of hips and knees is also common.

Contour changes include a decrease of fat in the body periphery and fat deposition over the abdomen and hips. The bony prominences become more marked.

For most older adults ROM testing proceeds as described earlier. ROM and muscle strength are much the same as with younger adults, provided there are no musculoskeletal illnesses or arthritic changes.

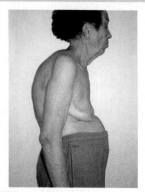

15.8 Postural changes with aging. (Lemmi and Lemmi, 2011.)

Normal Range of Findings	Abnormal Findings
Functional Assessment	
For those with advanced aging changes, arthritic changes, or musculoskeletal disability, perform a functional assessment for ADL. This applies the ROM and muscle strength assessments to the accomplishment of specific activities. You need to determine adequate and safe performance of functions essential for independent home life.	See Table 15.1 on p. 201.

Instructions to Person	Common Adaptation to Aging Changes	Instructions to Person	Common Adaptation to Aging Changes
1. Walk (with shoes on).	Shuffling pattern; swaying; arms out to help balance; broader base of support; person may watch feet.	4. Pick up object from floor.	Person often bends at waist instead of bending knees; holds furniture to support while bending and straightening.
2. Climb up stairs.	Person holds handrail; may haul body up with it; may lead with favored (stronger) leg.	5. Rise up from sitting in a chair.	Person uses arms to push off chair arms; upper trunk leans forward before body straightens; feet are planted wide in broad base of support.
3. Walk down stairs.	Holds handrail, sometimes with both hands. If the person is weak, he or she may descend sideways, lowering the weaker leg first. If the person is unsteady, he or she may watch feet.	6. Rise up from lying in bed.	May roll to one side, push with arms to lift up torso, grab bedside table to increase leverage.

HEALTH PROMOTION AND PATIENT TEACHING

Eat the rainbow. Choose colorful plates with green, red, orange, yellow, and purple foods. Starting in childhood, a diet rich in dark green and deep yellow vegetables (spinach, romaine lettuce, broccoli, carrots, sweet potatoes) and low in fried foods helps lower fat mass and promotes bone mass accrual.

Protect your bones by getting enough calcium and vitamin D. Women ages 50 years or younger need 1000 mg of calcium daily, and those over 50 need 1200 mg daily. Men age 70 years and younger need 1000 mg daily, increasing to 1200 mg daily for men over 70.

For bone health we recommend no more than 1 standard drink of alcohol daily for women and no more than 2 standard drinks per day for men. If you smoke, let's find a method to help you quit.

Physical activity delays or prevents bone loss; the more you do, the greater the benefit to your bones. If you are just getting started, aim for 2 or 3 days a week. Start easy so that you don't get hurt. Then work up to 30 minutes a day for 5 days a week.

All women should get a bone mineral density scan by DEXA by age 65 years; men by age 70 years.

Falls put you at risk of serious injury. Build your strength with an exercise program. Review your medicines with your provider to check which ones hurt your balance. Check your vision and hearing every year—eyes and ears keep you on your feet. Safety-proof your home: increase lighting, make stairs safe, remove trip hazards such as throw rugs, and install grab bars wherever needed (NCOA, 2017).

Summary Checklist: Musculoskeletal System

For each joint to be examined:
1. **Inspection:**
   Size and contour of joint
   Skin color and characteristics
2. **Palpation of joint area:**
   Skin
   Muscles
   Bony articulations
   Joint capsule

3. **ROM:**
   Active
   Passive (if there is limitation in active ROM)
4. **Muscle testing**

DOCUMENTATION

Sample Charting

SUBJECTIVE

States no joint pain, stiffness, swelling, or limitation. No muscle pain or weakness. No history of bone trauma or deformity. Able to manage all usual daily activities with no physical limitations. Occupation involves no musculoskeletal risk factors. Exercise pattern is brisk walk 1 mile 5×/week.

OBJECTIVE

Joints and muscles symmetric; no swelling, masses, deformity; normal spinal curvature. No tenderness to palpation of joints; no heat, swelling, or masses. Full ROM; movement smooth, no crepitus, no tenderness. Muscle strength—able to maintain flexion against resistance and without tenderness.

ASSESSMENT

Muscles and joints—healthy and functional

ABNORMAL FINDINGS

TABLE 15.1	Abnormalities Affecting Multiple Joints

Inflammatory Conditions

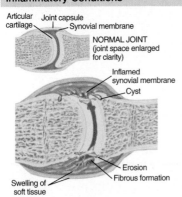

Degenerative Conditions

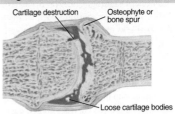

Rheumatoid Arthritis (RA)

This is a chronic autoimmune disease characterized by inflammation of synovial tissues and hyperplasia or swelling. This leads to fibrosis and to cartilage and bone destruction that limits motion and appears as deformity. Joint involvement is symmetric and bilateral, with heat, redness, swelling, and painful motion of affected joints. RA symptoms include fatigue, weakness, anorexia, weight loss, low-grade fever, and lymphadenopathy. RA carries increased cardiovascular risk of heart attack and stroke.

Osteoarthritis (OA) (Degenerative Joint Disease)

Localized, progressive disorder involving deterioration of articular cartilages (cushions between the ends of bones) and subchondral bone remodeling, synovial inflammation, and formation of new bone (osteophytes) at joint surfaces. Aging, female sex, and Caucasian ethnicity increase incidence. Obesity increases risk and progression of OA, especially in the knee (Hunter, 2015). Asymmetric joint involvement commonly affects hands, knees, hips, and lumbar and cervical segments of the spine. Affected joints have stiffness; swelling with hard, bony protuberances; pain with motion; and limitation of motion.

Continued

TABLE 15.1 | Abnormalities Affecting Multiple Joints—cont'd

Inflammatory Conditions	Degenerative Conditions
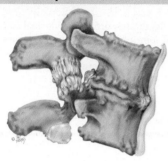	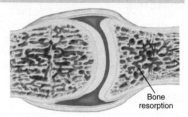 Bone resorption

Ankylosing Spondylitis (AS)

AS is chronic inflamed vertebrae (spondylitis) that in extreme form leads to bony fusion of vertebral joints (ankyloses). It affects the spine, pelvis, and thoracic cage, and is characterized by inflammatory back pain that is dull and deep in lower back or buttocks (Taurog, Chhabra, & Colbert, 2016). It also has morning back stiffness that lasts ≥30 minutes and decreases with activity, nighttime awakening with pain, age at onset ≤45 years. It affects males by a 2:1 ratio, beginning in late adolescence or early 20s. Spasm of paraspinal muscles pulls spine into forward flexion, obliterating cervical and lumbar curves. Thoracic curve exaggerated into single kyphotic rounding. Also includes flexion deformities of hips and knees as they compensate for spinal flexion.

Osteoporosis

Osteoporosis is a decrease in skeletal bone mass leading to low bone mineral density (BMD) and impaired bone quality. The weakened bone state increases risk for fractures, especially at the wrist, hip, and vertebrae. Occurs primarily in postmenopausal white women; also associated with smaller height and weight, younger age at menopause, lack of physical activity, and lack of estrogen in women.

See Illustration Credits for source information.

TABLE 15.2	Grading Muscle Strength		
Grade	**Description**	**Percent Normal**	**Assessment**
5	Full ROM against gravity, full resistance	100	Normal
4	Full ROM against gravity, some resistance	75	Good
3	Full ROM with gravity	50	Fair
2	Full ROM with gravity eliminated (passive motion)	25	Poor
1	Slight contraction	10	Trace
0	No contraction	0	Zero

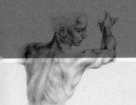

CHAPTER 16

Neurologic System

ANATOMY

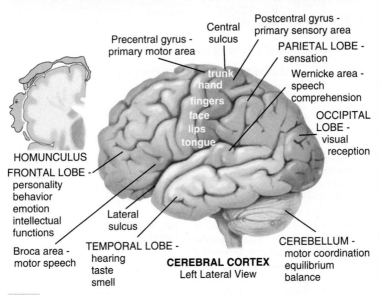

Central sulcus

Postcentral gyrus - primary sensory area

Precentral gyrus - primary motor area

PARIETAL LOBE - sensation

trunk
hand
fingers
face
lips
tongue

Wernicke area - speech comprehension

OCCIPITAL LOBE - visual reception

HOMUNCULUS

FRONTAL LOBE - personality behavior emotion intellectual functions

Lateral sulcus

Broca area - motor speech

TEMPORAL LOBE - hearing taste smell

CEREBRAL CORTEX
Left Lateral View

CEREBELLUM - motor coordination equilibrium balance

16.1 The lobes of the cerebral cortex and their specific functions.
(© Pat Thomas, 2006.)

The nervous system can be divided into two parts—central and peripheral. The **central nervous system** (CNS) includes the brain and spinal cord. The **peripheral nervous system** includes the 12 pairs of cranial nerves, the 31 pairs of spinal nerves, and all their branches. The peripheral nervous system carries sensory messages *to* the CNS from sensory receptors, motor messages *from* the CNS out to muscles and glands, and autonomic messages that govern the internal organs and blood vessels.

THE CENTRAL NERVOUS SYSTEM

The **cerebral cortex** is the outer layer of nerve cell bodies, also called *gray matter* (Fig. 16.1). The cerebral cortex is the center for humans' highest functions—governing thought, memory, reasoning, sensation, and voluntary movement.

203

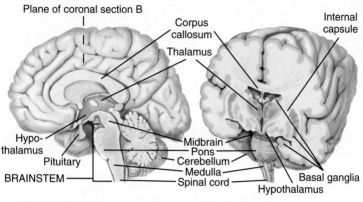

Plane of coronal section B

Corpus callosum

Thalamus

Internal capsule

Hypo-thalamus

Pituitary

BRAINSTEM

Midbrain
Pons
Cerebellum
Medulla
Spinal cord

Basal ganglia
Hypothalamus

A. Medial view of right hemisphere

B. Coronal section

COMPONENTS OF THE CENTRAL NERVOUS SYSTEM

16.2

(© Pat Thomas, 2006.)

Each half of the cerebrum is a **hemisphere**. Each hemisphere is divided into four **lobes**: frontal, parietal, temporal, and occipital.

The lobes have certain areas that mediate specific functions as labeled in Fig. 16.1. Damage to these specific cortical areas produces a corresponding loss of function: motor deficit, paralysis, loss of sensation, or impaired ability to understand and process language.

Beneath the cerebral cortex, the CNS has vital components (Fig. 16.2).

The **thalamus** is the main relay station for incoming sensory pathways and helps perform motor activities.

The **hypothalamus** controls temperature, sleep, emotions, autonomic activity, and the pituitary gland.

The **cerebellum** is concerned with motor coordination, equilibrium, and muscle tone.

The **midbrain** and **pons** contain motor neurons and motor and sensory tracts. The **medulla** contains fiber tracts and vital autonomic centers for respiration, heart, and gastrointestinal function.

The **spinal cord** is the main highway for ascending and descending fiber tracts that connect the brain to the spinal nerves, and it mediates reflexes.

THE PERIPHERAL NERVOUS SYSTEM

Cranial Nerves

Cranial nerves enter and exit the brain rather than the spinal cord (Fig. 16.3). The 12 pairs of cranial nerves supply primarily the head and neck, with the exception of the vagus nerve, which travels to the heart, respiratory muscles, stomach, and gallbladder.

Spinal Nerves

The 31 pairs of spinal nerves arise from the length of the spinal cord and supply the rest of the body (Fig. 16.4). They are named for the region of the spine from which they exit: 8 cervical, 12 thoracic, 5 lumbar, 5 sacral, and 1 coccygeal. They are "mixed" nerves because they contain both sensory and motor fibers.

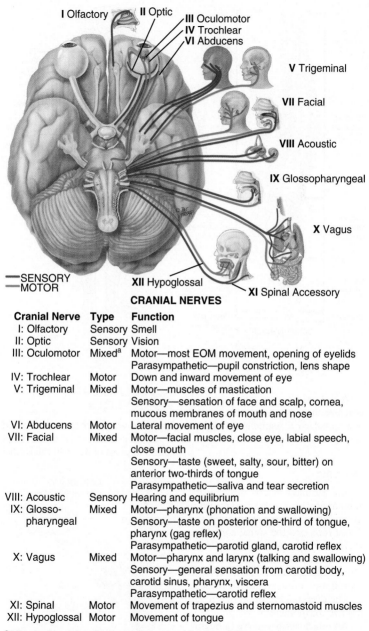

I Olfactory
II Optic
III Oculomotor
IV Trochlear
VI Abducens
V Trigeminal
VII Facial
VIII Acoustic
IX Glossopharyngeal
X Vagus
XII Hypoglossal
XI Spinal Accessory

SENSORY
MOTOR

CRANIAL NERVES

Cranial Nerve	Type	Function
I: Olfactory	Sensory	Smell
II: Optic	Sensory	Vision
III: Oculomotor	Mixed[a]	Motor—most EOM movement, opening of eyelids
		Parasympathetic—pupil constriction, lens shape
IV: Trochlear	Motor	Down and inward movement of eye
V: Trigeminal	Mixed	Motor—muscles of mastication
		Sensory—sensation of face and scalp, cornea, mucous membranes of mouth and nose
VI: Abducens	Motor	Lateral movement of eye
VII: Facial	Mixed	Motor—facial muscles, close eye, labial speech, close mouth
		Sensory—taste (sweet, salty, sour, bitter) on anterior two-thirds of tongue
		Parasympathetic—saliva and tear secretion
VIII: Acoustic	Sensory	Hearing and equilibrium
IX: Glosso-pharyngeal	Mixed	Motor—pharynx (phonation and swallowing)
		Sensory—taste on posterior one-third of tongue, pharynx (gag reflex)
		Parasympathetic—parotid gland, carotid reflex
X: Vagus	Mixed	Motor—pharynx and larynx (talking and swallowing)
		Sensory—general sensation from carotid body, carotid sinus, pharynx, viscera
		Parasympathetic—carotid reflex
XI: Spinal	Motor	Movement of trapezius and sternomastoid muscles
XII: Hypoglossal	Motor	Movement of tongue

[a]*Mixed* refers to a nerve carrying a combination of fibers: motor + sensory; motor + parasympathetic; or motor + sensory + parasympathetic.

16.3

(© Pat Thomas, 2006.)

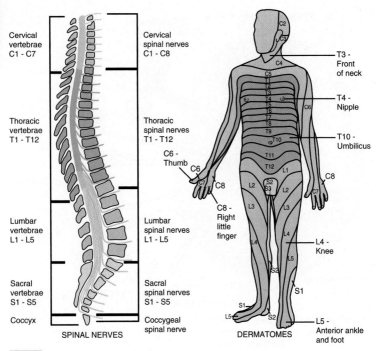

16.4 Spinal nerves and dermatomes.

A **dermatome** is a circumscribed skin area that is supplied mainly from one spinal cord segment through a particular spinal nerve.

Reflex Arc

In the simplest reflex the sensory afferent fibers carry the message from the receptor and travel through the dorsal root into the spinal cord (Fig. 16.5). They synapse in the cord with the motor neuron in the anterior horn. Motor efferent fibers leave via the ventral root and travel to the muscle.

The deep tendon or stretch reflex has five components:
1. An intact sensory nerve (afferent)
2. A functional synapse in the cord
3. An intact motor nerve fiber (efferent)
4. The neuromuscular junction
5. A competent muscle

CULTURE AND GENETICS

Stroke is an interruption of blood supply to the brain and is the 5th most common cause of death in the United

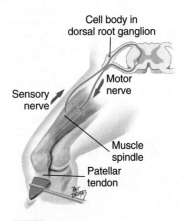

16.5 Reflex arc.

States (Mozaffarian et al., 2016). In the age-group of 45 to 64 years, African Americans have 2 to 3 times the risk of stroke as whites. About 40% of this risk is due to traditional stroke risk factors, especially high systolic BP (Mozaffarian et al., 2016). African Americans have a triple threat: (1) more likely to have high BP, (2) less likely to have their high BP controlled, and (3) suboptimal control yielding a stroke risk 3 times higher than in whites (Gutierrez & Williams, 2014). Metabolic syndrome (high blood glucose, dyslipidemia, obesity, hypertension) is 40% to 46% more prevalent among Mexican Americans than among non–Mexican-American whites and blacks; this is more evident in men than in women (Mozaffarian et al., 2016). These symptoms increase the risk for stroke. There also are disparities in access to care regarding stroke symptoms. Hispanic and Asian men and women are much less likely to use Emergency Medical Services transport to a hospital than are their white counterparts, and black women are less likely to use EMS than are white women (Mochari-Greenberger et al., 2015). Thus these groups experience longer delays before brain imaging and thrombolysis therapy.

SUBJECTIVE DATA

1. Headache (unusually frequent or severe)
2. Head injury or concussion
3. Dizziness (feeling light-headed or faint)/vertigo (feeling a rotational spinning)
4. Seizures
5. Tremors
6. Weakness or incoordination
7. Numbness or tingling
8. Difficulty swallowing
9. Difficulty speaking
10. Significant neurologic past history (stroke, spinal cord injury, meningitis or encephalitis, congenital defect, alcoholism)

OBJECTIVE DATA

PREPARATION

Perform a **screening** neurologic examination (items identified in following sections) on seemingly well people who have no significant subjective findings from the history.

Perform a **neurologic recheck** examination on people with demonstrated neurologic deficits who require periodic assessments (e.g., hospitalized people or those in extended care), using the examination sequence beginning on p. 221.

EQUIPMENT NEEDED

Penlight
Tongue blade
Cotton swab
Cotton ball
Tuning fork (128 or 256 Hz)
Percussion hammer

Normal Range of Findings	Abnormal Findings

Mental Status

Assess level of consciousness (see Chapter 2 and examination sequence on p. 9).

Test Cranial Nerves

Cranial Nerve II—Optic Nerve

Test visual acuity and test visual fields by confrontation. When indicated, use the ophthalmoscope to examine the ocular fundus (see Chapter 7).

Visual field loss (see Table 15.5, p. 310, in Jarvis: *Physical Examination and Health Assessment,* 8th ed.).

Papilledema with increased intracranial pressure; optic atrophy (see Table 15.9, p. 314, in Jarvis: *Physical Examination and Health Assessment,* 8th ed.).

Cranial Nerves III, IV, and VI—Oculomotor, Trochlear, and Abducens Nerves

Palpebral fissures are usually equal in width or nearly so.

Ptosis (drooping) with myasthenia gravis, dysfunction of cranial nerve III, or Horner syndrome (see Table 7.2, p. 78).

For CN III, check pupils for size, regularity, equality, light reaction, and accommodation (see Chapter 7). The pupils are normally equal, round, react to light promptly, and react to accommodation (PERRLA).

Assess extraocular movements by the cardinal positions of gaze (see Chapter 7).

Nystagmus is a back-and-forth oscillation of the eyes. Endpoint nystagmus, a few beats of horizontal nystagmus at extreme lateral gaze, occurs normally. Assess any other nystagmus carefully.

Unequal size, constricted pupils, dilated pupils, or no response to light (see Table 7.3, p. 80).

Deviated gaze or limited movement.

Cranial Nerve V—Trigeminal Nerve

Motor Function. Palpate the temporal and masseter muscles as the person clenches the teeth. Muscles should feel equally strong on both sides. Try to separate the jaws by pushing down on the chin; normally you cannot.

Decreased strength on one or both sides.

Pain with clenching of teeth.

Normal Range of Findings	Abnormal Findings

Sensory Function. With the person's eyes closed, test light touch sensation by touching a cotton wisp to these designated areas on the person's face: forehead, cheeks, and chin. Ask the person to say "now" whenever the touch is felt.

Decreased or unequal sensation. With a stroke, sensation is lost in face and body on the opposite side of the lesion.

Cranial Nerve VII—Facial Nerve

Motor Function. Note mobility and facial symmetry as the person responds to these requests: smile, frown, close eyes tightly (against your attempt to open them), lift eyebrows, show teeth, and puff cheeks.

Muscle weakness shows by loss of the nasolabial fold, drooping of one side of the face, lower eyelid sagging, and escape of air from only one puffed cheek when both are pressed in.

Cranial Nerve VIII—Acoustic

Test hearing by person's ability to hear normal conversation and the whispered voice test (see Chapter 8).

Cranial Nerves IX and X— Glossopharyngeal and Vagus

Depress with a tongue blade and note movement as the person says "ahh"; uvula and soft palate should rise in the midline, and tonsillar pillars move medially.

Absence or asymmetry of soft palate movement may occur after a stroke; swallowing then increases risk of aspiration.

Cranial Nerve XI—Spinal Accessory

Check strength of neck muscles by asking person to turn head forcibly against your resistance at side of chin and to shrug shoulders against resistance. Both sides should feel equally strong.

Atrophy of neck muscles. Muscle weakness or paralysis occurs with a stroke or injury to a peripheral nerve.

Cranial Nerve XII—Hypoglossal

Ask person to stick out tongue; should protrude in the midline. Ask person to say, "light, tight, dynamite"; lingual speech should be clear and distinct.

Fasciculations. Tongue deviates to side when stroke affects the hypoglossal nerve.

Inspect and Palpate the Motor System

Muscles

Size. Muscle groups should be within the normal size limits for age

Normal Range of Findings	Abnormal Findings

and should be symmetric bilaterally. When muscles in the extremities appear asymmetric, measure each in centimeters and record the difference. A difference of 1 cm or less is not significant. Note that it is difficult to assess muscle mass in very obese people.

Atrophy—Abnormally small muscle with a wasted appearance; occurs with disuse, injury, lower motor neuron disease, and muscle disease.

Hypertrophy—Increased size and strength; occurs with isometric exercise.

Strength. Test homologous muscles simultaneously (see Chapter 15).

Paralysis—Loss of motor power, (see Table 16.1, p. 227).

Cerebellar Function

Gait. Observe as the person walks 10 to 20 feet, turns, and returns to the starting point. Normally the gait is smooth, rhythmic, and effortless; the opposing arm swing is coordinated; turns are smooth. The step length is about 15 inches from heel to heel.

Stiff, immobile posture. Staggering or reeling. Wide base of support.
Lack of arm swing or rigid arms.

Ask the person to walk a straight line in a heel-to-toe fashion (tandem walking) (Fig. 16.6). This decreases the base of support and accentuates any problem with coordination. Normally the person can walk straight and stay balanced.

Unequal rhythm of steps. Slapping of foot. Scraping of toe of shoe.

Ataxia—Uncoordinated or unsteady gait.
Crooked line of walk.
Widens base to maintain balance.
Staggering, reeling, loss of balance.

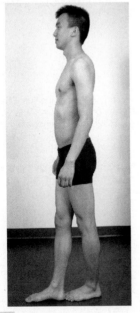

16.6 Walk heel-to-toe.

Normal Range of Findings	Abnormal Findings

Romberg Test. Ask the person to stand with feet together and arms at the sides. Once in a stable position, ask the person to close the eyes and hold the position (Fig. 16.7). Wait about 20 seconds. Normally a person can maintain posture and balance, although there may be slight swaying. (Stand close to catch the person in case he or she falls.)

An ataxia that did not appear with regular gait may now appear.

Swaying, falling, widening of base of feet to avoid falling.

Positive Romberg sign is loss of balance increased by closing of the eyes. It occurs with cerebellar ataxia (multiple sclerosis, alcohol intoxication), loss of proprioception, and loss of vestibular function.

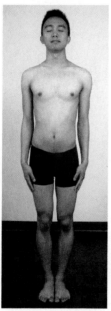

16.7 Romberg test.

Ask the person to perform a shallow knee bend or to hop in place, first on one leg and then the other. This demonstrates normal position sense, muscle strength, and cerebellar function. Note that some individuals cannot hop because of aging or obesity.

Assess the Sensory System

Make sure the person is alert, cooperative, and comfortable and has an adequate attention span; otherwise you may get misleading and invalid results.

Normal Range of Findings	Abnormal Findings

Routine screening procedures include testing superficial pain, light touch, vibration in a few distal locations.

The person's eyes should be closed during each test. Take time to explain what will be happening and exactly how you expect the person to respond.

Superficial Pain

Twist and break a tongue blade lengthwise, forming a sharp point at the fractured end and a dull spot at the rounded end. Lightly apply the sharp point and the dull end to the person's body in a random, unpredictable order (Fig. 16.8). Ask the person to say "sharp" or "dull," depending on the sensation felt. (Note that the sharp edge is used to test for pain; the dull edge is used as a general test of the person's responses.) Alternatively break a cotton swab in half, forming a sharp point and using the dull spot at the cotton end.

Hypoalgesia—Decreased pain sensation.

Analgesia—Absent pain sensation.
Hyperalgesia—Increased pain sensation.

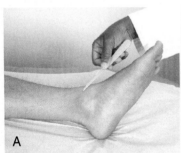 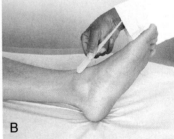

16.8   Test superficial pain.

Let at least 2 seconds elapse between each stimulus to avoid *summation*. With summation, frequent consecutive stimuli are perceived as one strong stimulus.

Normal Range of Findings	Abnormal Findings

Light Touch

Apply a wisp of cotton to the skin. Stretch a cotton ball to make a long end and brush it over the skin in a random order of sites and at irregular intervals. Ask the person to say "now" or "yes" when touch is felt. Compare symmetric points.

Hypoesthesia—Decreased touch sensation.
Anesthesia—Absent touch sensation.
Hyperesthesia—Increased touch sensation.

Vibration

Strike a low-pitched tuning fork on the heel of your hand and hold the base on a bony surface of the fingers and great toe (Fig. 16.9). Ask the person to indicate when the vibration starts and stops. The normal response is vibration or a buzzing sensation on these distal areas. If no vibrations are felt, move proximally and test ulnar processes, ankles, patellae, and iliac crests. Compare the right side to the left. If you find a deficit, note whether it is gradual or abrupt.

Unable to feel vibration; states that vibration stops when fork is still vibrating.
Loss of vibration sense occurs with peripheral neuropathy, e.g., diabetes and alcoholism. This is often the first sensation lost.

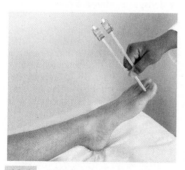

16.9   Vibration.

Normal Range of Findings	Abnormal Findings

Test the Reflexes

Stretch or Deep Tendon Reflexes (DTRs)

For an adequate response the limb should be relaxed, and the muscle partially stretched. Stimulate the reflex by directing a short, snappy blow of the reflex hammer onto the insertion tendon of the muscle. Strike a brief, well-aimed blow and bounce up promptly; do not let the hammer rest on the tendon. Use the pointed end of the reflex hammer when aiming at a smaller target such as your thumb on the tendon site; use the flat end when the target is wider or to diffuse the impact and prevent pain.

Use just enough force to get a response. Compare right and left sides; the responses should be equal. The reflex response is graded on a four-point scale:

4 + Very brisk, hyperactive with clonus; indicates disease
3 + Brisker than average; may indicate disease
2 + Average; normal
1 + Diminished; low normal
0 No response

Clonus is a set of short, jerking contractions of the same muscle following the hammer blow.

Hyperreflexia is the exaggerated reflex seen when the monosynaptic reflex arc is released from the influence of higher cortical levels. This occurs with CNS upper motor neuron lesions, e.g., after a stroke.

Hyporeflexia, which is the absence of a reflex, is a lower motor neuron problem. It occurs with interruption of sensory afferents or destruction of motor efferents and anterior horn cells, e.g., spinal cord injury.

Biceps Reflex (C5 to C6). Support the person's forearm on yours; this position relaxes and partially flexes his or her arm. Place your thumb on the biceps tendon and strike a blow on your thumb. You can both feel and see the normal response, which is flexion of the forearm (Fig. 16.10).

Normal Range of Findings	Abnormal Findings

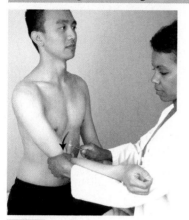

16.10   Biceps reflex.

Triceps Reflex (C7 to C8). Tell the person to let the arm "just go dead" as you suspend it by holding the upper arm. Strike the triceps tendon directly just above the elbow (Fig. 16.11). The normal response is extension of the forearm. Alternatively hold the person's wrist across the chest to flex the arm at the elbow and tap the tendon.

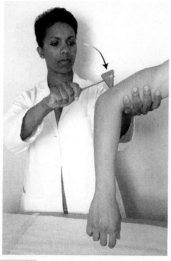

16.11   Triceps reflex.

Normal Range of Findings

Abnormal Findings

Patellar Reflex ("Knee Jerk") (L2 to L4). Let the lower legs dangle freely to flex the knee and stretch the tendons. Strike the tendon directly just below the patella (Fig. 16.12). Extension of the lower leg is the expected response. Also you can feel the contraction of the quadriceps.

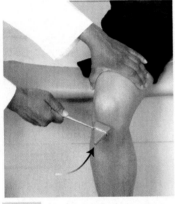

16.12 Patellar reflex.

Achilles Reflex ("Ankle Jerk") (L5 to S2). Position the person with the knee flexed and the hip externally rotated. Hold the foot in dorsiflexion and strike the Achilles tendon directly (Fig. 16.13). Feel the normal response as the foot plantar flexes against your hand.

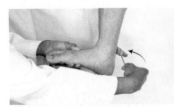

16.13 Achilles reflex.

Normal Range of Findings	Abnormal Findings

Plantar Reflex (L4 to S2). With the end of the reflex hammer, draw a light stroke up the lateral side of the sole and across the ball of the foot, like an upside-down J (Fig. 16.14, *A*). The normal response is plantar flexion of the toes and sometimes of the entire foot.

Except in infancy, the abnormal response is dorsiflexion of the big toe and fanning of all toes, which is a **positive Babinski sign**. This occurs with upper motor neuron disease of the pyramidal tract (see Fig. 16.14, *B*).

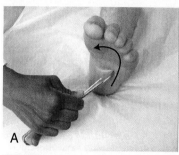
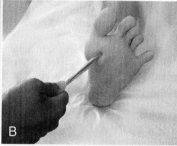

16.14 **A,** Plantar reflex. **B,** Babinski sign.

 DEVELOPMENTAL COMPETENCE

Infants (Birth to 12 Months)

Assessment includes noting that milestones you normally would expect for each month have indeed been achieved and that the early, more primitive reflexes are eliminated from the baby's repertory when they are supposed to be.

Observe spontaneous motor activity for smoothness and symmetry. Smoothness of movement suggests proper cerebellar function, as does the coordination involved in sucking and swallowing. To screen gross and fine motor coordination, use the Denver-II Developmental Screening Test with its age-specific developmental milestones.

Check the muscle tone necessary for head control. With the baby supine and holding the wrists, pull the infant into a sitting position and note head control. The newborn holds the head

Failure to attain a skill by expected time.
Persistence of reflex behavior beyond the normal time.

Delay in motor activity occurs with brain damage, mental retardation, peripheral neuromuscular damage, prolonged illness, parental neglect, and environmental disaster.

Normal Range of Findings	Abnormal Findings
in almost the same plane as the body; the head balances briefly when the baby reaches a sitting position and then flops forward. (Even a premature infant shows some head flexion.) At 4 months of age the head stays in line with the body and does not flop.	Because development progresses in a cephalocaudal direction, head lag is an early sign of brain damage. After 6 months of age any baby with failure to hold the head in midline when sitting should be referred.

Reflexes have a predictable time-table of appearance and departure. For the screening examination, check the rooting, grasp, Babinski, tonic neck, and Moro reflexes.

Rooting Reflex. Brush the infant's cheek near the mouth. He or she normally turns the head toward that side and opens the mouth. The reflex appears at birth and disappears within 3 or 4 months.

Palmar Grasp. Offer your finger and note tight grasp of all the baby's fingers. Sucking enhances grasp. You can often pull baby to a sitting position from grasp. The reflex is present at birth, is strongest at 1 to 2 months, and disappears at 3 to 4 months.

Babinski Reflex. Stroke your finger up the lateral edge and across the ball of the infant's foot. Note fanning of toes (positive Babinski reflex; Fig. 16.15). The reflex is present at birth and disappears (changes to the adult response) by 24 months of age (variable).

The reflex is absent with brain damage and with local muscle or nerve injury.

Persistence of the reflex after 4 months of age occurs with frontal lobe lesion.

Positive Babinski reflex after 2 or 2½ years of age occurs with pyramidal tract disease.

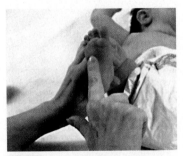

16.15 Babinski reflex.

Normal Range of Findings	Abnormal Findings

Tonic Neck Reflex. With the baby supine, relaxed, or sleeping, turn the head to one side with the chin over the shoulder. Note ipsilateral extension of the arm and leg and flexion of the opposite arm and leg; this is the "fencing" position. If you turn the infant's head to the opposite side, positions reverse (Fig. 16.16). The reflex appears by 2 to 3 months, decreases at 3 to 4 months, and disappears by 4 to 6 months.

Persistence later in infancy occurs with brain damage.

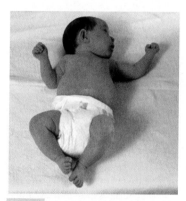

16.16 Tonic neck reflex.

Moro Reflex. Startle the infant by jarring the crib, making a loud noise, or supporting the head and back in a semi-sitting position and quickly lowering the infant to 30 degrees. The baby looks as if he or she is hugging a tree; there is symmetric abduction and extension of the arms and legs, fanning fingers, and curling the index finger and thumb to a C position. The infant then brings in both arms and legs (Fig. 16.17). The reflex is present at birth and disappears at 1 to 4 months.

Absence of the Moro reflex in the newborn or persistence after 5 months of age indicates severe CNS injury.

Absence of movement in one arm occurs with fracture of the humerus or clavicle and with brachial nerve palsy.

Absence in one leg occurs with a lower spinal cord problem or a dislocated hip.

A hyperactive Moro reflex occurs with tetany or CNS infection.

Normal Range of Findings	Abnormal Findings

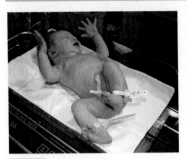

16.17   Moro reflex.

The Aging Adult

Use the same examination as used with younger adults. Be aware that some aging adults show a slower response to your requests, especially to those calling for coordination of movements.

Any decrease in muscle bulk is most apparent in the hand, as seen by guttering between the metacarpals. These dorsal hand muscles often look wasted, even with no apparent arthropathy. The grip strength remains relatively good.

Senile tremors occasionally occur. These benign tremors include an intention tremor of the hands, head nodding (as if saying yes or no), and tongue protrusion. There is no associated rigidity.

The gait may be slower, may be more deliberate, and may deviate slightly from a midline path compared with the gait in the younger person.

After 65 years of age loss of the sensation of vibration at the ankle malleolus is common and usually accompanied by loss of the ankle jerk. Tactile sensation may be impaired. The aging person may need stronger stimuli for light touch and especially pain.

The deep tendon reflexes are less brisk. Those in the upper extremities are usually present, but the ankle jerks

Hand muscle atrophy is worsened with disuse and degenerative arthropathy.

Distinguish senile tremors from tremors of parkinsonism. The latter include rigidity, slowness, and weakness of voluntary movement.

Absence of a rhythmic, reciprocal gait pattern is seen in parkinsonism and hemiparesis.

Note any difference in sensation between the right and left sides, which may indicate a neurologic deficit.

Normal Range of Findings	Abnormal Findings

are commonly lost. Knee jerks may be lost, but this occurs less often.

The plantar reflex may be absent or difficult to interpret. Often you do not see a definite normal flexor response; however, you should still consider a definite extensor response to be abnormal.

Hospital Neurologic Checks

Some hospitalized people have head trauma or a neurologic deficit due to a systemic disease process. These people must be monitored closely for any improvement or deterioration in neurologic status and for any indication of increasing intracranial pressure. Use an abbreviation of the neurologic examination in the following sequence:

1. Level of consciousness
2. Motor function
3. Pupillary response
4. Vital signs

Level of Consciousness. A *change* in the level of consciousness is the single most important factor in this examination. It is the earliest and most sensitive index of change in neurologic status. Note the ease of *arousal* and the state of awareness, or *orientation*. Assess orientation by asking questions about:

- Person—Own name, occupation, names of workers around person, his or her occupation
- Place—Where person is, nature of building, city, state
- Time—Day of week, month, year

Vary the questions during repeat assessments so the person is not merely memorizing answers.

Note the quality and content of the verbal response and articulation, fluency, manner of thinking, and any deficit in language comprehension or production (see Chapter 2).

A person is fully alert when his or her eyes open at your approach or

Signs of increasing intracranial pressure signal impending cerebral disaster and death and require early and prompt intervention.

A change in consciousness may be subtle. Note any decreasing level of consciousness, disorientation, memory loss, uncooperative behavior, or even complacency in a previously combative person.

Review Table 2.1, Levels of Consciousness, p. 13.

Normal Range of Findings	Abnormal Findings

spontaneously; when he or she is oriented to person, place, and time; and when he or she is able to follow verbal commands appropriately.

If the person is not fully alert, increase the amount of stimulus used in this order:

1. Name called
2. Light touch on person's arm
3. Vigorous shake of shoulder
4. Pain applied (pinch nail bed, pinch trapezius muscle, rub your knuckles on the person's sternum)

Record the stimulus used and the person's response to it.

Motor Function. Check the voluntary movement of each extremity by giving the person specific commands. (This procedure also tests level of consciousness by noting the person's ability to follow commands.)

Ask the person to lift the eyebrows, frown, and bare the teeth. Note symmetric facial movements and bilateral nasolabial folds (cranial nerve VII).

Check upper arm strength by checking hand grasps. Ask the person to squeeze your fingers. Offer your two fingers, one on top of the other, so that a strong hand grasp does not hurt your knuckles.

A weak grip occurs with upper motor neuron and lower motor neuron disease and with arthritis.

Check lower extremities by asking the person to do straight leg raises. Ask the person to lift one leg at a time straight up off the bed. Full strength allows the leg to be lifted 90 degrees. If multiple trauma, pain, or equipment precludes this motion, ask the person to push one foot at a time against your hand's resistance, "like putting your foot on the gas pedal of your car."

For the person with decreased level of consciousness, note if movement occurs spontaneously and as a result of noxious stimuli such as pain or suctioning. An attempt to push your

Any abnormal posturing, decorticate rigidity, or decerebrate rigidity indicates diffuse brain injury (see Table 24.10, p. 680, in Jarvis: *Physical Examination and Health Assessment,* 8th ed.).

Normal Range of Findings	Abnormal Findings

hand away after such stimuli is called *localizing* and characterized as purposeful movement.

Pupillary Response. Note the size, shape, and symmetry of both pupils. Shine a light into each pupil and note the direct and consensual light reflex. Both pupils should constrict briskly. (Allow for the effects of any medication that could affect pupil size and reactivity.) When recording, pupil size is best expressed in millimeters. Tape a millimeter scale onto a tongue blade and hold it next to the person's eyes for the most accurate measurement (Fig. 16.18).

In a brain-injured person, a sudden, unilateral, dilated, and nonreactive pupil is ominous. Cranial nerve III runs parallel to the brainstem. When increasing intracranial pressure pushes the brainstem down (uncal herniation), it puts pressure on cranial nerve III, causing pupil dilation.

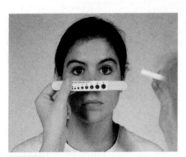

16.18   Measure   pupil   size   in millimeters.

Vital Signs. Measure the temperature, pulse, respiration, and blood pressure as often as the person's condition warrants. Although they are vital to the overall assessment of the critically ill person, pulse and blood pressure are notoriously unreliable parameters of CNS deficit. Any changes are late consequences of rising intracranial pressure.

The Glasgow Coma Scale (GCS). The GCS is an objective assessment that defines the level of consciousness by giving it a numeric value (Fig. 16.19).

Signs of increasing intracranial pressure, the *Cushing reflex:*
Blood pressure—Sudden elevation with widening pulse pressure.
Pulse—Decreased rate, slow and bounding.

Normal Range of Findings	Abnormal Findings

GLASGOW COMA SCALE						
EYE OPENING RESPONSE		**MOTOR RESPONSE**		**VERBAL RESPONSE**		
Spontaneous	4	*wiggle your fingers* — Obeys verbal command	6	*what year is it?* [correct response] — Oriented X3 -appropriate	5	
To speech	3	Localizes pain	5	*what year is it?* 1962 — Conversation confused	4	
		Flexion - withdrawal	4	*what year is it?* after lunch — Speech inappropriate	3	
To pain	2	Flexion - abnormal	3	*what year is it?* aawagga — Speech incomprehensible	2	Normal total 15
		Extension - abnormal	2			
No response	1	No response	1	No response	1	
	SUB-TOTAL	– – – → plus	SUB-TOTAL	– – – → plus	SUB-TOTAL	**TOTAL SCORE**

16.19

(Images © Pat Thomas, 2014.)

The scale is divided into three areas: eye opening, motor response, and verbal response. Each area is rated separately, and a number is given for the person's best response. The three numbers are added; the total score reflects the brain's functional level. A fully alert, normal person has a score of 15. Serial assessments can be plotted on a graph to illustrate visually whether the person is stable, improving, or deteriorating.

See Table 16.2, p. 228.

A score of 7 or less reflects coma.

HEALTH PROMOTION AND PATIENT TEACHING

Know about Stroke. Know the Signs so you can Act in Time. A stroke or brain attack occurs when blood flow is interrupted to a part of the brain. Because stroke symptoms usually do not hurt, many people ignore them or delay seeking medical attention. Paying attention to these symptoms can save lives.

Common symptoms of stroke (NINDS, 2017) include **sudden** onset of the following:

- Weakness or numbness in the face, arms, or legs, especially when it is on one side of the body.

- Confusion, trouble speaking or understanding.
- Changes in vision, such as blurry vision or partial or complete loss of vision in one or both eyes.
- Trouble walking, dizziness, loss of balance or coordination.
- Severe headache with no reason or explanation.

The F.A.S.T. plan (NINDS, 2017) is the easy way to remember the sudden signs of stroke:

- F = Face drooping
- A = Arm weakness
- S = Speech difficulty
- T = Time to call 9-1-1

Vaccination can decrease the risk of herpes zoster (HZ), or shingles, in older adults. HZ shows as a painful red blistered rash along a nerve route on one side of the body. It often is followed by a chronic lingering pain along the nerve (postherpetic neuralgia). However, HZ does not have to happen. The herpes zoster vaccine reduces the risk of shingles and is recommended for those over 60 years. The vaccine comes in one dose as a shot, and can be given in a provider's office or pharmacy.

Summary Checklist: Neurologic Screening Examination

1. **Mental status (level of consciousness)**
2. **Cranial nerves:**
   II—Optic
   III, IV, VI—Pupil response and extraocular muscles
   V—Jaw muscles and facial sensation
   VII—Facial mobility
3. **Motor function:**
   Gait and balance
   Knee flexion—Hop or shallow knee bend
4. **Sensory function:**
   Superficial sharp and light touch—Arms and legs
   Vibration—Arms and legs
5. **Reflexes:**
   Biceps
   Triceps
   Patellar
   Achilles
   Plantar

DOCUMENTATION

Sample Charting

SUBJECTIVE

No unusually frequent or severe headaches; no head injury, dizziness or vertigo, seizures, or tremors. No weakness, numbness or tingling, difficulty swallowing or speaking. No past history of stroke, spinal cord injury, meningitis, or alcohol disorder.

OBJECTIVE

Mental Status: Appearance, behavior, and speech appropriate; alert and oriented to person, place, and time; recent and remote memory intact.

Cranial Nerves:
> II: Vision 20/20 left eye, 20/20 right eye; peripheral fields intact by confrontation; fundi normal.
>
> III, IV, VI: EOMs intact, no ptosis or nystagmus; pupils equal, round, react to light and accommodation (PERRLA).
>
> V: Sensation intact and equal bilaterally; jaw strength equal bilaterally.
>
> VII: Facial muscles intact and symmetric.
>
> VIII: Hearing—whispered words heard bilaterally.
>
> IX, X: Swallowing intact, uvula rises in midline on phonation.
>
> XI: Shoulder shrug, head movement intact and equal bilaterally.
>
> XII: Tongue protrudes midline, no tremors.

Motor: No atrophy, weakness, or tremors. Gait smooth and coordinated, able to tandem walk, negative Romberg.

Sensory: Sharp and dull sensation, light touch, vibration intact.

Reflexes: DTRs 2+ and = bilaterally with downgoing toes.

ASSESSMENT

Neurologic system intact, healthy function

TABLE 16.1	Abnormal Muscle Movement

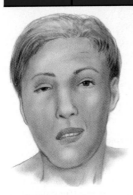

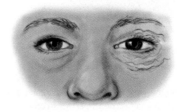

Paralysis

Decreased or loss of motor power due to problem with motor nerve or muscle fibers. Causes: acute—trauma, spinal cord injury, brain attack, poliomyelitis, polyneuritis, Bell palsy; chronic—muscular dystrophy, diabetic neuropathy, multiple sclerosis; episodic—myasthenia gravis.

Fasciculation

Rapid, continuous twitching of resting muscle that can be seen or palpated. Types: fine—occurs with lower motor neuron disease, associated with atrophy and weakness; coarse—occurs with cold exposure or fatigue and is not significant.

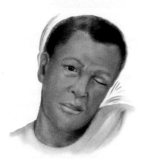

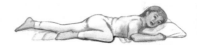

Tic

Involuntary, compulsive, repetitive twitching of a muscle group, e.g., wink, grimace, head movement, shoulder shrug; from a neurologic cause, e.g., tardive dyskinesias, Tourette syndrome; or psychogenic cause, e.g., habit tic.

Myoclonus

Rapid, sudden jerk at fairly regular intervals. A hiccup is a myoclonus of diaphragm. Single myoclonic arm or leg jerk is normal when the person is falling asleep; myoclonic jerks are severe with grand mal seizures.

Tremor (see following page)

Involuntary contraction of opposing muscle groups. Results in rhythmic, back-and-forth movement of one or more joints. May occur at rest or with voluntary movement. Tremors may be slow (3 to 6 per second) or rapid (10 to 20 per second).

Continued

TABLE 16.1 Abnormal Muscle Movement—cont'd

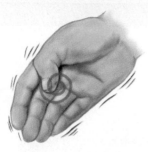

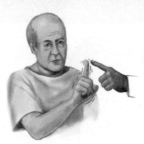

Rest Tremor

Occurs when muscles are quiet and supported against gravity. Coarse and slow (3 to 6 per second); partly or completely disappears with voluntary movement, e.g., "pill rolling" tremor of parkinsonism, with thumb and opposing fingers.

Intention Tremor

Rate varies; worse with voluntary movement toward a visual target. Occurs with cerebellar disease and multiple sclerosis. Essential tremor (familial)—a type of intention tremor; most common tremor with older people. Benign (no associated disease) but causes emotional stress.

TABLE 16.2 Abnormal Postures

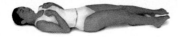

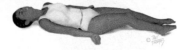

Decorticate Rigidity

Upper extremities—flexion of arm, wrist, and figures; adduction of arm (i.e., tight against thorax). Lower extremities—extension, internal rotation, plantar flexion. This indicates hemispheric lesion of cerebral cortex.

Decerebrate Rigidity

Upper extremities stiffly extended, adducted; internal rotation, palms pronated. Lower extremities stiffly extended, plantar flexion; teeth clenched; hyperextended back. More ominous than decorticate rigidity; indicates lesion in brainstem at midbrain or upper pons.

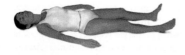

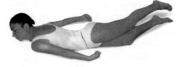

Flaccid Quadriplegia

Complete loss of muscle tone and paralysis of all four extremities, indicating completely nonfunctional brainstem.

Opisthotonos

Prolonged arching of back, with head and heels bent backward; indicates meningeal irritation.

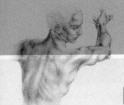

CHAPTER 17

Male Genitourinary System

Male Genital Structures

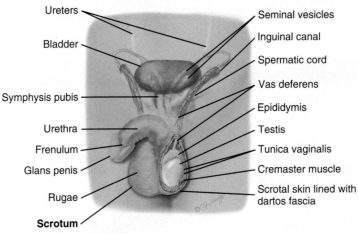

Ureters
Bladder
Symphysis pubis
Urethra
Frenulum
Glans penis
Rugae
Scrotum

Seminal vesicles
Inguinal canal
Spermatic cord
Vas deferens
Epididymis
Testis
Tunica vaginalis
Cremaster muscle
Scrotal skin lined with dartos fascia

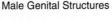

17.1   The male genital structures.   (© Pat Thomas, 2010.)

The **male genitalia** include the penis and scrotum externally and the testis, epididymis, and vas deferens internally (Fig. 17.1). The accessory glandular structures (prostate, seminal vesicles) are discussed in Chapter 19.

The **urethra** traverses the penis, and its meatus forms a slit at the glans tip. The **scrotum** is a loose sac, which is a continuation of the abdominal wall. In each scrotal half is a **testis,** which produces sperm. The testis has a solid oval shape and is about 4 to 5 cm long by 3 cm wide in adults.

The testis is capped by the **epididymis,** which is a markedly coiled duct system that stores sperm. The epididymis is continuous with a muscular duct,

the **vas deferens**, which approximates with other vessels to form the **spermatic cord**. The spermatic cord runs through the inguinal canal into the abdomen.

Puberty is beginning earlier in boys than in previous U.S. studies—now at average age of 9 years for African-American boys and 10 years for Caucasians and Hispanics (Herman-Giddens et al., 2012). The first sign is enlargement of the testes. Next pubic hair appears, and then penis size increases. The stages of development are documented in Tanner's sexual maturity ratings (SMR) (see Table 25.1 in Jarvis: *Physical Examination and Health Assessment*, 8th ed., p. 686)

SUBJECTIVE DATA

1. Frequency, urgency, and nocturia
2. Dysuria (pain or burning with urination)
3. Hesitancy and straining
4. Urine color (cloudy or hematuria)
5. Genitourinary history (kidney disease, kidney stones, flank pain, urinary tract infections, prostate trouble)
6. Penis—Pain, lesion, discharge
7. Scrotum—Pain, lumps
8. Patient-centered care—HPV vaccination, perform testicular self-examination
9. Sexual activity, condom and contraceptive use
10. Sexually transmitted infection (STI) contact

OBJECTIVE DATA

PREPARATION

Position the male standing with undershorts down and appropriate draping. The examiner should be sitting. Alternatively the male may be supine for the first part of the examination and then stand during the hernia check.

EQUIPMENT NEEDED

Urine screen for chlamydia and gonorrhea
Gloves—Wear gloves during every male genitalia examination
Flashlight (occasionally)

Normal Range of Findings	Abnormal Findings
Inspect and Palpate the Penis	
The skin normally looks wrinkled, hairless, and without lesions.	Generalized swelling. Inflammation. Lesions: nodules, solitary ulcer (chancre), grouped vesicles or superficial ulcers, wartlike papules (see Table 25.4, p. 705, in Jarvis: *Physical Examination and Health Assessment,* 8th ed.).
The glans looks smooth and without lesions. Ask the uncircumcised male to retract the foreskin or you may retract it. It should move easily. After inspection slide the foreskin back to the original position.	Phimosis—Foreskin is advanced and fixed, so it cannot be retracted. Paraphimosis—Foreskin is retracted and fixed, so it cannot be returned to original position.
The urethral meatus is positioned just about centrally on the glans (Fig. 17.2).	Hypospadias—Ventral location of meatus. Epispadias—Dorsal location of meatus (see Table 25.5, p. 707, in Jarvis: *Physical Examination and Health Assessment,* 8th ed.).

Normal Range of Findings	Abnormal Findings

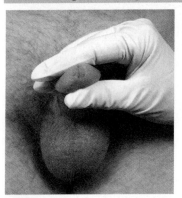

17.2

Compress the glans anteroposteriorly between your thumb and forefinger. The edge of the meatus should appear pink, smooth, and without discharge.

Stricture—Narrowed opening.
Edges that are red, everted, and edematous, along with purulent discharge, suggest urethritis (see Table 25.3, p. 704, in Jarvis: *Physical Examination and Health Assessment,* 8th ed.).

Palpate the shaft between your thumb and first two fingers. The penis normally feels smooth, semi-firm, and nontender.

Nodule; induration.
Tenderness.

Inspect and Palpate the Scrotum

Scrotal size varies with ambient room temperature. Asymmetry is normal, with the left scrotal half lower than the right. Lift the sac to inspect the posterior surface. Normally there are no scrotal lesions except for the commonly found sebaceous cysts. These are yellowish, 1-cm nodules that are firm, nontender, and often multiple.

Scrotal swelling (edema) may be taut and pitting. This occurs with heart failure, renal failure, and local inflammation.
Lesions.
Inflammation.

Palpate each scrotal half between your thumb and first two fingers. Testes normally feel oval, firm and rubbery, and smooth and equal bilaterally. They are freely movable and slightly tender to moderate pressure. Each epididymis normally feels discrete, softer than the testis, smooth, and nontender.

Absent testis—May be a temporary migration or true cryptorchidism (see Table 17.1, p. 236).
Atrophied testes—Small and soft.
Fixed testes.
Nodules on testes or epididymides.
Marked tenderness.

Normal Range of Findings	Abnormal Findings
Between your thumb and forefinger palpate each spermatic cord along its length, from the epididymis up to the external inguinal ring. It should feel smooth and nontender.	Thickened cord. Soft, swollen, and tortuous cord—See varicocele, Table 17.1, p. 237.
Normally there are no other scrotal contents. If you do find a mass, note: • Is there any tenderness? • Is the mass distal or proximal to the testis? • Can you place your fingers over it? • Does it reduce when the person lies down? • Can you auscultate bowel sounds over it?	Abnormalities in the scrotum—Hernia, tumor, orchitis, epididymitis, hydrocele, spermatocele, varicocele (see Table 17.1, pp. 238-239).

Inspect and Palpate for Hernia

Inspect the inguinal region for a bulge as the male stands and as he strains down. Normally there is none.	Bulge at external inguinal ring or femoral canal. (A hernia may be present but easily reduced and appears only intermittently with an increase in intra-abdominal pressure.)
Palpate the inguinal canal (Fig. 17.3). Ask the patient to shift his weight onto the unexamined leg. Place your index finger low on the scrotal half. Palpate up the length of the spermatic cord, invaginating the scrotal skin as you go, to the external inguinal ring. The inguinal ring feels like a triangular, slitlike opening, and it may or may not admit your finger. If it admits your finger, gently insert it into the canal and ask the person to bear down. Normally you will feel no change. Repeat the procedure on the other side.	Palpable herniating mass bumps your fingertip or pushes against the side of your finger (see Table 25.7, p. 711, in Jarvis: *Physical Examination and Health Assessment,* 8th ed.).

External inguinal ring

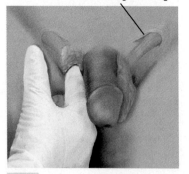

17.3 Palpate for inguinal hernia.

Normal Range of Findings	Abnormal Findings
Palpate the femoral area for a bulge. Normally you feel none.	

Inguinal Lymph Nodes

Palpate the horizontal chain along the groin inferior to the inguinal ligament and the vertical chain along the upper inner thigh.

On occasion it is normal to palpate an isolated node. It feels small (<1 cm), soft, discrete, and movable.

Enlarged, hard, matted, fixed nodes.

Testicular Self-Examination (TSE)

Encourage self-care by teaching each male (from 13 to 14 years old through adulthood) to examine his own testicles every month.

The incidence of testicular cancer is rare but most commonly occurs in young men ages 15 to 35.

A testicular tumor has no early symptoms. If it is detected early by palpation and treated, the prognosis is much improved. Early detection is enhanced if the person is familiar with the normal consistency of his testes. Phrase the teaching something like this:

A good time to examine the testicles is during the shower or bath when your hands and scrotum are warm. Cold hands stimulate a muscular (cremasteric) reflex, retracting the scrotal contents. The procedure is simple. Hold the scrotum in the palm of your hand and gently feel each testicle with your thumb and first two fingers. If it hurts, you are using too much pressure. The testicle is egg shaped and movable. It feels rubbery with a smooth surface, like a hard-boiled egg. The epididymis is on top and behind the testicle; it feels a bit softer. If you notice a firm, painless lump; a hard area; or an overall enlarged testicle, call your doctor for a further check.

 DEVELOPMENTAL COMPETENCE

Infants and Children

Palpate the scrotum and testes. Take care not to elicit the cremasteric reflex that pulls the testes up into the inguinal canal. (1) Keep your hands warm and palpate from the external inguinal ring down. (2) Block the inguinal canals with the thumb and forefinger of your other hand to prevent the testes from retracting (Fig. 17.4).

Normal Range of Findings	Abnormal Findings

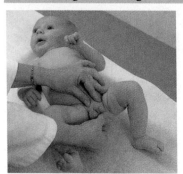

17.4 Palpate infant testes.

Normally the testes are descended and are equal in size bilaterally (1.5 to 2 cm until puberty). Once palpated, testes are considered descended, even if they have retracted momentarily.

If the scrotal half feels empty, search for the testes along the inguinal canal and try to milk them down. Ask the toddler or child to squat with the knees flexed up: this pressure may force the testes down.

Migratory testes (physiologic cryptorchidism) are common because of the strength of the cremasteric reflex and the small mass of the prepubertal testes. Note that the affected side has a normally developed scrotum and that the testis can be milked down. These testes descend at puberty and are normal.

Cryptorchidism—Undescended testes (those that have never descended). Undescended testes are common in premature infants. They occur in 3% to 4% of term infants, although most have descended by 3 months of age. The age at which a child should be referred differs among physicians (see Table 17.1, p. 236).

With true cryptorchidism the scrotum is atrophic.

The Aging Adult

In the older male you may note thinner, graying pubic hair and a decreased size of the penis. The size of the testes may be decreased, and they may feel less firm. The scrotal sac is pendulous, with less rugae. The scrotal skin may become excoriated if the man continually sits on it.

Summary Checklist: Male Genitourinary System

1. Inspect and palpate the penis.
2. Inspect and palpate the scrotum.
3. If a mass exists, note associated signs.
4. Palpate for an inguinal hernia.
5. Palpate the inguinal lymph nodes.
6. Teach testicular self-examination.

HEALTH PROMOTION AND PATIENT TEACHING

We have described the technique of testicular self-examination during your exam. Now let's discuss the benefits and risks and how often you may want to perform the exam yourself. The benefits of TSE involve becoming comfortable with your own body and being able to follow up with your provider in a timely manner if you do find a lump or thickening. Most lumps are not cancerous, but when a lump is cancerous, early detection and treatment have the highest rates of survival, almost 100%. The risks involved with TSE if you ever find a lump include additional office visits, testing and radiologic imaging, and possible anxiety while the tests are conducted. The American Cancer Society has no official recommendation on regular performance of TSE. One interesting study was done, however—a cost-utility study (Aberger et al., 2014). This study found a 2.4 to 1 cost-benefit ratio for early detection of testicular cancer versus finding and treating cancer at advanced stages (Aberger et al., 2014). *So we have this information to discuss and your personal decision.*

DOCUMENTATION

Sample Charting

SUBJECTIVE

Urinates 4 or 5 times/day, clear, straw-colored. No nocturia, dysuria, or hesitancy. No pain, lesions, or discharge from penis. Does not do testicular self-examination. No history of genitourinary disease. Sexually active in a monogamous relationship. Sexual life satisfactory to self and partner. Uses birth control via barrier method (partner uses diaphragm). No known STI contact.

OBJECTIVE

No lesions, inflammation, or discharge from penis. Scrotum—testes descended, symmetric, no masses. No inguinal hernia.

ASSESSMENT

Genital structures normal and healthy

ABNORMAL FINDINGS

TABLE 17.1	Scrotal Abnormalities	
Disorder	Clinical Findings	Discussion
Absent Testis **Cryptorchidism** 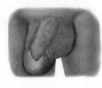	S: Empty scrotal half O: Inspection—In true maldescent, atrophic scrotum on affected side Palpation—No testis A: Absent testis	True cryptorchidism—Testes have never descended. Incidence at birth is 3% to 4%; one-half of these descend in first month. Incidence with premature infants is 30%. True undescended testes have a histologic change by 6 years, causing decreased spermatogenesis and infertility.
Small Testis 	S: (None) O: Palpation—Small and soft (rarely may be firm) A: Small testis	Small and soft (<3.5 cm) indicates atrophy from cirrhosis, hypopituitarism, estrogen therapy, or orchitis. Small and firm (<2 cm) occurs with Klinefelter syndrome (hypogonadism).
Testicular Torsion 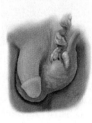	S: Excruciating pain in testicle of sudden onset, often during sleep or after trauma; may have lower abdominal pain, nausea and vomiting, no fever O: Inspection—Red, swollen scrotum; one testis (usually left) higher due to rotation and shortening Palpation—Cord feels thick, swollen, tender; epididymis may be anterior; cremasteric reflex is absent on side of torsion	Sudden twisting of spermatic cord. Occurs in late childhood, early adolescence. Usually occurs on the left side. Faulty anchoring of testis on wall of scrotum allows testis to rotate. The anterior part of the testis rotates medially toward the other testis. Blood supply is cut off, resulting in ischemia and engorgement. This is an emergency requiring surgery; testis can become gangrenous in a few hours.

S = Subjective data; O = objective data; A = assessment.   *Continued*

TABLE 17.1	Scrotal Abnormalities—cont'd	
Disorder	**Clinical Findings**	**Discussion**
Epididymitis 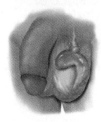	S: Severe pain of sudden onset in scrotum, relieved by elevation (a positive Prehn sign); also rapid swelling, fever O: Inspection—Enlarged scrotum; reddened Palpation—Exquisitely tender; epididymis enlarged, indurated, hard to distinguish from testis. Overlying scrotal skin may be thick, edematous Laboratory—White blood cells and bacteria in urine A: Tender swelling of epididymis	Acute infection of epididymis commonly caused by prostatitis, after prostatectomy because of trauma of urethral instrumentation, or due to chlamydia, gonorrhea, or other bacterial infection. Often difficult to distinguish between epididymitis and testicular torsion.
Spermatic Cord Varicocele 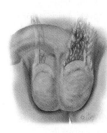	S: Dull pain; constant pulling or dragging feeling; or may be asymptomatic O: Inspection—Usually no sign; may show bluish color through light scrotal skin Palpation—When standing, feel soft, irregular mass posterior to and above testis; collapses when supine, refills when upright; feels distinctive, like a "bag of worms"; testis on the side of the varicocele may be smaller because of impaired circulation A: Soft mass on spermatic cord	A varicocele is dilated, tortuous internal spermatic veins due to incompetent valves, which permit reflux of blood. Most often on left side, perhaps because left spermatic vein is longer and inserts at a right angle into left renal vein. Common in young males. Screen at early adolescence; early treatment important to prevent potential infertility when an adult. Treatment is relatively easy; surgical ligation of spermatic vein.

Continued

TABLE 17.1	Scrotal Abnormalities—cont'd	
Disorder	**Clinical Findings**	**Discussion**
Spermatocele 	S: Painless, usually found on examination O: Inspection—Transilluminates higher in the scrotum than a hydrocele, and the sperm may fluoresce Palpation—Round, freely movable mass lying above and behind testis; if large, feels like a third testis A: Free cystic mass on epididymis	Retention cyst in epididymis. Cause unclear but may be obstruction of tubules. Filled with thin, milky fluid that contains sperm. Most spermatoceles are small (<1 cm); occasionally they may be larger and then mistaken for hydrocele.
Early Testicular Tumor 	S: Painless, found on examination O: Palpation—Firm nodule or harder than normal section of testicle A: Solitary nodule	Most testicular tumors occur between the ages of 18 and 35; most are malignant. Occur in whites; rare in blacks, Mexican Americans, and Asians. Must biopsy to confirm. Most important risk factor is undescended testis, even those surgically corrected. Early detection aids prognosis, but practice of TSE is low.
Diffuse Tumor 	S: Enlarging testis (most common symptom); when enlarged, has feel of increased weight O: Inspection—Enlarged, does not transilluminate Palpation—Enlarged, smooth, ovoid, firm Important—Firm palpation does not cause usual sickening discomfort as with normal testis A: Nontender swelling of testis	Diffuse tumor maintains shape of testis.

Continued

TABLE 17.1	Scrotal Abnormalities—cont'd	
Disorder	**Clinical Findings**	**Discussion**
Hydrocele 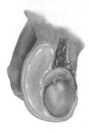	S: Painless swelling, may complain of weight and bulk in scrotum O: Inspection—Enlarged, mass transilluminates with a pink or red glow (in contrast to a hernia) Palpation—Nontender mass; able to get fingers above mass (in contrast to scrotal hernia) A: Nontender swelling of testis	Cystic. Circumscribed collection of serous fluid in tunica vaginalis surrounding testis. May occur following epididymitis, trauma, hernia, tumor of testis, or spontaneously in the newborn.
Scrotal Hernia 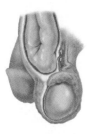	S: Swelling, may have pain with straining O: Inspection—Enlarged, may reduce when supine, does not transilluminate Palpation—Soft mushy mass; palpating fingers cannot get above mass; mass is distinct from normal testicle A: Nontender swelling of scrotum	Scrotal hernia usually caused by indirect inguinal hernia.
Orchitis 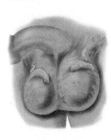	S: Acute or moderate pain of sudden onset, swollen testis, feeling of weight, fever O: Inspection—Enlarged, edematous, reddened; does not transilluminate Palpation—Swollen, congested, tense, and tender; hard to distinguish testis from epididymis A: Tender swelling of testis	Acute inflammation of testis. Most common cause is mumps; can occur with any infectious disease. May have associated hydrocele that does transilluminate.

Continued

TABLE 17.1	Scrotal Abnormalities—cont'd	
Disorder	**Clinical Findings**	**Discussion**
Scrotal Edema	S: Tenderness O: Inspection—Enlarged; may be reddened (with local irritation) Palpation—Taut with pitting; probably unable to feel scrotal contents A: Scrotal edema	Accompanies marked edema in lower half of body, e.g., heart failure, renal failure, portal vein obstruction. Occurs with local inflammation: epididymitis, torsion of spermatic cord. Obstruction of inguinal lymphatics produces lymphedema of scrotum.

Images © Pat Thomas, 2006.

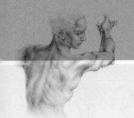
Female Genitourinary System

ANATOMY

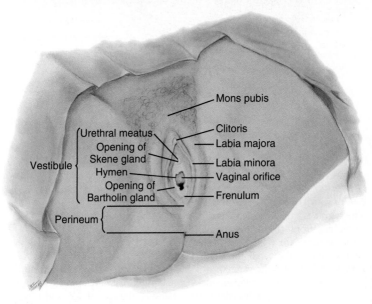

18.1 The external genitalia.

External Genitalia

The external female genitalia are called the **vulva** or pudendum (Fig. 18.1). The **mons pubis** is a round, firm pad of adipose tissue covering the symphysis pubis. The labia majora and labia minora encircle a space termed the **vestibule.** Within this space the urethral meatus appears as a dimple 2.5 cm posterior to the clitoris. The **clitoris** is a small, pea-shaped erectile body that is highly sensitive to tactile stimulation.

The vaginal orifice is posterior to the urethral meatus. On either side and posterior to the vaginal orifice are the two **Bartholin glands,** which secrete a clear lubricating mucus during intercourse.

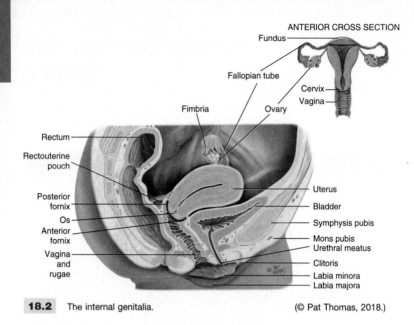

ANTERIOR CROSS SECTION

Fundus

Fallopian tube

Cervix

Vagina

Fimbria

Ovary

Rectum

Rectouterine pouch

Posterior fornix

Os

Anterior fornix

Vagina and rugae

Uterus

Bladder

Symphysis pubis

Mons pubis

Urethral meatus

Clitoris

Labia minora

Labia majora

18.2 The internal genitalia. (© Pat Thomas, 2018.)

Internal Genitalia

The **vagina** is a flattened tubular canal extending from the orifice up and backward into the pelvis (Fig. 18.2). At the end of the canal the uterine **cervix** projects into the vagina.

The **uterus** is a pear-shaped, thick-walled, muscular organ. It is flattened anteroposteriorly, measuring 5.5 to 8 cm long × 3.5 to 4 cm wide and 2 to 2.5 cm thick, is movable, and usually tilts forward.

The **fallopian tubes** are two trumpet-shaped, pliable tubes, 10 cm in length, extending from the uterine fundus laterally to the brim of the pelvis, with their ends near the ovaries. Each **ovary** is oval, 3 cm long × 2 cm wide by 1 cm thick, and serves to develop ova (eggs) and the female hormones.

DEVELOPMENTAL COMPETENCE

The first signs of puberty are breast and pubic hair development, beginning between the ages of 8½ and 13 years. These signs are usually concurrent, but it is not abnormal if they do not develop together. They take about 3 years to complete.

Menarche occurs during the latter half of this sequence, just after the peak of growth velocity.

Tanner's table on the five stages of pubic hair development is helpful in teaching girls the expected sequence of sexual development (Table 18.1).

TABLE 18.1	Sex Maturity Rating (SMR) in Girls
Stage	Description
1	Preadolescent. No pubic hair. Mons and labia covered with fine vellus hair as on abdomen.
2	Growth sparse and mostly on labia. Long, downy hair; slightly pigmented; straight or only slightly curly.
3	Growth sparse and spreading over mons pubis. Hair is darker, coarser, curlier.
4	Hair is adult in type but over smaller area: none on medial thigh.
5	Adult in type and pattern; inverse triangle. Also on medial thigh surface.

Adapted from Tanner, J.M. (1962). *Growth at adolescence*, Oxford, England: Blackwell Scientific.

SUBJECTIVE DATA

1. Menstrual history; last menstrual period (LMP), age at menarche, cycle, duration
2. Obstetric history
   Gravida—Number of pregnancies
   Para—Number of births
   Interrupted pregnancies (elective abortions, spontaneous miscarriages)
3. Menopause
4. Patient-centered care—HPV vaccine, gynecologic checkup, Pap test
5. Acute pelvic pain
6. Urinary symptoms
   Frequency, urgency, dysuria
7. Vaginal discharge—Color, characteristics
8. Sexual activity, contraceptive use, condom use
9. Sexually transmitted infection (STI)
10. STI risk reduction taught

OBJECTIVE DATA

PREPARATION

Initially for the health history the woman should be sitting up.

For the examination, help her into the lithotomy position, with the body supine, feet in stirrups and knees apart, and buttocks at edge of examining table. The arms should be at the woman's sides or across the chest, not over the head, because this position only tightens the abdominal muscles. Elevate head of table to 45 degrees.

Drape the woman fully, covering the stomach, knees, and legs; but be sure to push down the drape between the woman's legs so you can see her face.

You can help the woman relax, decrease her anxiety, and retain a sense of control by using these measures: have her empty the bladder before the examination; elevate her head and shoulders to maintain eye contact; place the stirrups so the legs are not abducted too far; explain each step in the examination before you do it; assure the woman that she can say "stop" at any point should she feel any discomfort; use a gentle, firm touch with gradual movements; communicate throughout the examination; maintain a dialogue to share information.

EQUIPMENT NEEDED

Urine (first catch) specimen for STI screening

Assemble the following items before helping the woman into position. Arrange within easy reach.

Gloves—Wear gloves during every female genitalia examination

Goose-necked lamp with a strong light

Vaginal speculum of appropriate size

Graves speculum—For adult women in varying lengths and widths

Pedersen speculum—Narrow blades for young or postmenopausal women with a narrowed introitus

Large cotton-tipped applicators (rectal swabs)

Materials for cytologic study:
  Liquid-based cytology vial
  Endocervical brush (cytobrush)
  Specimen container for gonococcus/chlamydia

Lubricant

Normal Range of Findings	Abnormal Findings

Inspect the External Genitalia

The skin color is even.

Hair distribution is in the usual female pattern of an inverted triangle, although it may normally trail up the abdomen toward the umbilicus.

Labia majora are normally symmetric, plump, and well formed. In the nulliparous woman labia meet in the midline; following a vaginal delivery the labia are gaping and slightly shriveled.

Consider delayed puberty if no pubic hair or breast development has occurred by age 13.

Nits or lice at base of pubic hair.

Swelling.

Normal Range of Findings	Abnormal Findings

There should be no lesions, except for occasional sebaceous cysts. These are yellowish, 1-cm nodules that are firm, nontender, and often multiple.

Excoriation. Nodules. Rash/lesions. Refer suspicious red, white, or pigmented lesion for evaluation and biopsy (see Table 27.2, p. 756, in Jarvis: *Physical Examination and Health Assessment,* 8th ed.).

With your gloved hand, separate the labia majora to inspect the clitoris.

Labia minora are dark pink and moist, usually symmetric.

Urethral opening appears stellate or slitlike and is midline.

Vaginal opening, or introitus, may appear as a narrow vertical slit or as a larger opening.

Perineum is smooth. A well-healed episiotomy scar, midline or mediolateral, may be present after a vaginal birth.

Anus has coarse skin of increased pigmentation (see Chapter 19 for assessment).

Enlarged clitoris.
Inflammation.

Polyp.

Rash or lesions.
Foul-smelling; irritating; or yellow, white, or gray discharge.

Palpate Glands

Assess Bartholin glands. Palpate the posterior parts of the labia majora with your index finger in the vagina and your thumb outside (Fig. 18.3). The labia normally feel soft and homogeneous.

Swelling.
Pain on palpation.
Discharge from duct opening.

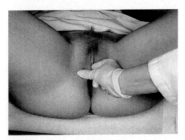

18.3   Palpate labia majora.

Assess the Support of Pelvic Musculature

Palpate the perineum. It normally feels thick, smooth, and muscular in

Tenderness.
Paper-thin perineum.

Normal Range of Findings	Abnormal Findings

nulliparous women and thin and rigid in multiparous women.

Using your index and middle fingers, separate the vaginal orifice and ask the woman to strain down. There normally is no bulging of vaginal walls or urinary incontinence.

Bulging of the vaginal wall indicates cystocele, rectocele, or uterine prolapse (see Table 27.3, p. 758, in Jarvis: *Physical Examination and Health Assessment,* 8th ed.).

Urinary incontinence.

Internal Genitalia

Speculum Examination

Select the proper-size speculum; warm and lubricate it. Evidence shows that applying a small amount (dime size) of water-soluble gel lubricant on the outer inferior blade increases patient comfort and yields no more unsatisfactory slides than does water-only lubricant (Lin et al., 2014).

Hold the speculum in your left hand with the index and middle fingers surrounding the blades and your thumb under the thumbscrew. This prevents the blades from opening painfully during insertion. With your right index and middle fingers, push the introitus down and open to relax the pubococcygeal muscle (Fig. 18.4).

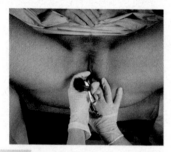

18.4   Insert vaginal speculum.

Tilt the width of the blades obliquely and insert the speculum past your right fingers, applying any pressure downward. This avoids pressure on the anterior vaginal wall and on the sensitive urethra above it.

Normal Range of Findings	Abnormal Findings

Ease insertion by asking the woman to bear down. This method relaxes the perineal muscles and opens the introitus.

As the blades pass your right fingers, withdraw your fingers. Now change the hand holding the speculum to your right hand and turn the width of the blades horizontally. Continue to insert in a 45-degree angle downward toward the small of the woman's back. This matches the natural slope of the vagina.

After the blades are fully inserted, open them by squeezing the handles together (Fig. 18.5). The cervix should be in full view. Lock the blades open by tightening the thumbscrew.

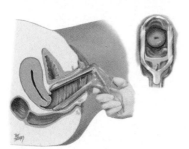

18.5 Open speculum blades and view cervix.

Inspect the Cervix and Its Os

The color of the cervical mucosa is pink and even. During the second month of pregnancy it looks blue (Chadwick sign), and after menopause it is pale.

Redness, inflammation.
Pallor with anemia.
Cyanosis other than with pregnancy.

(See Table 27.4, p. 758, in Jarvis: *Physical Examination and Health Assessment,* 8th ed.)

The position is midline, either anterior or posterior. It projects 1 to 3 cm into the vagina.

The size—Diameter is 2.5 cm (1 inch).

The Os—Small and round in nulliparous women. In parous women it is a horizontal irregular slit and may show healed lacerations on the sides.

The surface is normally smooth.

Surface reddened, granular, and any lesion (see erosion, polyp, carcinoma, Table 27.4, p. 759, in Jarvis: *Physical Examination and Health Assessment,* 8th ed.).

Normal Range of Findings	Abnormal Findings
Cervical secretions—Depending on the day of the menstrual cycle, secretions may be clear and thin or thick, opaque, and stringy. They are always odorless and nonirritating.	Foul-smelling; irritating; or yellow, green, white, or gray discharge (see Table 27.5, p. 760, in Jarvis: *Physical Examination and Health Assessment,* 8th ed.).

If secretions are copious, swab the area with a thick-tipped rectal swab. This method sponges away secretions, giving you a better view of the structures.

Obtain Cervical Test and Cultures

The Pap test screens for cervical cancer. Instruct the woman not to douche or have intercourse within 24 hours before collecting the specimens. The test requires three specimens:

Vaginal Pool. Gently rub the blunt end of cytobrush over the vaginal wall under and lateral to the cervix. Gently stir the end into the liquid collection vial. If the mucosa is very dry (as in a postmenopausal woman), moisten a sterile swab with normal saline to collect this specimen.

Cervical Scrape. Use the cytobrush to gather cells on the cervix—especially on the transitional zone that extends onto the cervix in adolescents.

Endocervical Cells. Insert a cytobrush into the os and rotate it 720 degrees in *ONE* direction (Fig. 18.6). Then dip into the liquid collection vial.

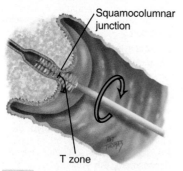

Squamocolumnar junction

T zone

18.6 Endocervical specimen.

Normal Range of Findings	Abnormal Findings

Inspect the Vaginal Wall

Loosen the thumbscrew but continue to hold the speculum blades open. Slowly withdraw the speculum, rotating it as you go, to fully inspect the vaginal wall. Normally the wall looks pink, deeply rugated, moist, and smooth, and it is free of inflammation or lesions. Normal discharge is thin and clear or opaque and stringy but always is odorless.

When the blade ends are near the vaginal opening, let them close, but be careful not to pinch the mucosa or catch any hairs. Turn the blades obliquely to avoid stretching the opening. Clean the metal speculum and place it in a sterilizing and disinfecting solution; discard the plastic variety. Discard your gloves and wash hands.

Reddened.
Pallor before menopause.
Lesions; refer any suspicious red, white, or pigmented lesion for biopsy.
Vaginal discharge—Thick; any gray, green-yellow, white, or foul-smelling discharge.
(See Table 27.5, p. 761, in Jarvis: *Physical Examination and Health Assessment,* 8th ed.)

Bimanual Examination

Rise to a stand and have the woman remain in the lithotomy position. Glove and lubricate the first two fingers of your intravaginal hand. Insert your fingers into the vagina, with any pressure directed posteriorly.

Use both hands to palpate the internal genitalia to assess their location, size, and mobility and screen for any tenderness or mass. One hand is on the abdomen while the other (often the dominant, more sensitive hand) inserts two fingers into the vagina.

Palpate the Internal Genitalia

Palpate the vaginal wall. It normally feels smooth and has no area of induration or tenderness.

Locate the cervix in the midline, often near the anterior vaginal wall. Note these characteristics of a normal cervix:

Nodule.
Tenderness.

Normal Range of Findings	Abnormal Findings

Consistency—Feels smooth and firm, like the consistency of the tip of the nose. It softens and feels velvety at 5 to 6 weeks of pregnancy (Goodell sign).

Hard with malignancy.
Nodular.

Contour is evenly rounded.

Mobility—With a finger on either side, move the cervix gently from side to side. Normally this produces no pain (Fig. 18.7).

Irregular.
Immobile with malignancy.
Painful with inflammation or ectopic pregnancy.

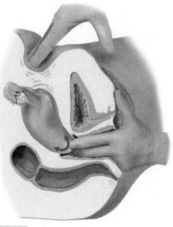

18.7 Palpate the cervix.

Palpate all around the fornices; the wall should feel smooth.

Nodular.
Irregular.

Next use your abdominal hand to push the pelvic organs closer for your intravaginal fingers to palpate. Place your hand midway between the umbilicus and the symphysis; push down in a slow, firm manner, with the fingers together and slightly flexed.

With your intravaginal fingers in the anterior fornix, assess the uterus. Determine the position, or *version,* of the uterus. In many women the uterus is anteverted; you palpate it at the level of the pubis with the cervix pointing posteriorly. Two other positions normally occur (midposition and

Normal Range of Findings	Abnormal Findings

retroverted), as well as two aspects of flexion, where the long axis of the uterus is not straight but flexed (for illustration, see Fig. 27.19, p. 748, in Jarvis: *Physical Examination and Health Assessment,* 8th ed.).

Palpate the uterine wall with your fingers in the fornices. It normally feels firm and smooth, with the contour of the fundus rounded. It softens during pregnancy. Bounce the uterus gently between your abdominal and intravaginal hand. It should be freely movable and nontender.

Move both hands to the right to explore the adnexa. Place your abdominal hand on the lower quadrant just inside the anterior iliac spine with your intravaginal fingers in the lateral fornix (Fig. 18.8). Push the abdominal hand in and try to capture the ovary. You often cannot feel the ovary. When you can, it normally feels smooth, firm, and almond-shaped; it is highly movable, sliding through the fingers. It is slightly sensitive but not painful. The fallopian tube normally is not palpable. There should be no other mass or pulsation.

Enlarged uterus (see Table 27.6, p. 762, in Jarvis: *Physical Examination and Health Assessment*, 8th ed.).
Lateral displacement.
Nodular mass. Irregular, asymmetric. Fixed.
Tenderness.

Enlarged adnexa.
Nodular.
Immobile.
Markedly tender.
Mass.

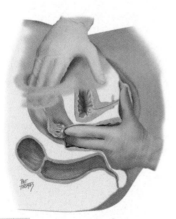

18.8 Palpate the adnexa.

Pulsation or a palpable fallopian tube suggests ectopic pregnancy and warrants immediate referral (see Table 27.7, p. 763, in Jarvis; *Physical Examination and Health Assessment*, 8th ed.).

Normal Range of Findings	Abnormal Findings

Move to the left to palpate the other side. Then withdraw your hand and check secretions on the fingers before discarding the glove. Normal secretions are clear or cloudy and odorless.

A note of caution: Normal adnexal structures are often not palpable. To be safe, any mass that you cannot positively identify as a normal structure should be considered abnormal. Refer the woman to a gynecologist.

Rectovaginal Examination

Use this technique to assess the rectovaginal septum, posterior uterine wall, cul-de-sac, and rectum. Lubricate your first two fingers. Tell the woman that this may feel uncomfortable and will mimic the feeling of moving her bowels. Ask her to bear down as you insert your index finger into the vagina and your middle finger gently into the rectum (Fig. 18.9).

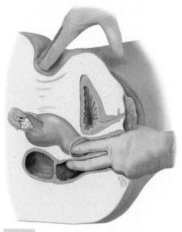

18.9 Rectovaginal palpation.

While pushing with the abdominal hand, repeat the steps of the bimanual examination. Try to keep the intravaginal finger on the cervix so the intrarectal finger does not mistake the cervix for a mass.

Normal Range of Findings	Abnormal Findings
The rectovaginal septum should feel smooth, thin, firm, and pliable.	Nodular.
	Thickened.

The rectovaginal pouch, or cul-de-sac, is a potential space and usually not palpated.

The uterine wall and fundus feel firm and smooth.

Rotate the intrarectal finger to check the rectal wall and anal sphincter tone. (See Chapter 19 for assessment of the anus and rectum.) Check your gloved finger as you withdraw; test any adherent stool for occult blood.

Give the woman tissues to wipe the area and help her up. Remind her to slide her hips back from the table edge before sitting up so she does not fall.

DEVELOPMENTAL COMPETENCE

The Pregnant Woman

The external genitalia show hyperemia of the perineum and vulva because of increased vascularity. Varicose veins may be visible in the labia or legs. Hemorrhoids may show around the anus. Both are caused by interruption in venous return from the pressure of the fetus.

Internally the walls of the vagina appear violet or blue because of hyperemia. The vaginal walls are deeply rugated, and the vaginal mucosa is thickened. The cervix looks blue and feels velvety and softer than in the nonpregnant state, making it a bit more difficult to differentiate from the vaginal walls.

During bimanual examination the isthmus of the uterus feels softer and is more easily compressed between your two hands (Hegar sign). The fundus balloons between your two hands; it feels connected to, but distinct from,

Normal Range of Findings	Abnormal Findings
the cervix because the isthmus is so soft. Search the adnexal area carefully during early pregnancy. Normally the adnexal structures are not palpable.	An ectopic pregnancy has serious consequences (see Table 27.7, p. 763, in Jarvis: *Physical Examination and Health Assessment,* 8th ed.).

The Aging Adult

Natural lubrication is decreased; to avoid a painful examination, take care to lubricate instruments and the examining hand adequately. Use the Pedersen speculum with its narrower, flatter blades.

Menopause and the resulting decrease in estrogen production cause numerous physical changes. Pubic hair gradually decreases, becoming thin and sparse in later years. Fat deposits decrease, leaving the mons pubis smaller and the labia flatter. Clitoris size also decreases after age 60.

Internally the rugae of the vaginal walls decrease, and the walls look pale pink because of the thinned epithelium. The cervix shrinks and looks pale and glistening. It may retract, appearing to be flush with the vaginal wall. In some older women it is hard to distinguish the cervix from the surrounding vaginal mucosa. Alternately the cervix may protrude into the vagina if the uterus has prolapsed.

With the bimanual examination the uterus feels smaller and firmer, and the ovaries are not normally palpable.

Summary Checklist: Female Genitourinary System

1. Inspect external genitalia.
2. Palpate labia and Bartholin glands.
3. Using vaginal speculum, inspect cervix and vagina.
4. Obtain specimens for cytologic study.
5. Perform bimanual examination: cervix, uterus, adnexa.
6. Perform rectovaginal examination.
7. Test stool for occult blood.

HEALTH PROMOTION AND PATIENT TEACHING

The Adolescent

Ensure confidentiality and a private time to talk. Then address these talking points. (For suggested phrasing, see Jarvis: *Physical Examination and Health Assessment*, 8th ed., p. 753.)

Recommend HPV vaccination with completion of series.

Prepare for possible sexual activity. If not ready, strategies to postpone. If ready, use of condoms.

If in committed heterosexual relationship, needs teaching and products to prevent unintended pregnancy and STIs.

Gender identity; sexual identity. Address openness to explore teen's feelings.

Use of alcohol and drugs, especially tied to coercive sex or unplanned sex.

Physical safety in family and sexual relationships.

Cyberbullying, bullying behaviors at school.

DOCUMENTATION

Sample Charting

SUBJECTIVE

Menarche age 12 years, cycle usually q 28 days, duration 5 days, flow moderate, no dysmenorrhea, LMP April 3. Grav 0/Para 0/Ab 0. Gyne checkup and last Pap test 1 year PTA, negative.

No urinary problems, no irritating or foul-smelling vaginal discharge, no sores or lesions, no history pelvic surgery. Satisfied with sexual relationship with husband, uses vaginal diaphragm for birth control, no plans for pregnancy at this time. Not aware of any STI contact to herself or husband.

OBJECTIVE

External genitalia: No swelling, lesions, or discharge. No urethral swelling or discharge.
Internal: Vaginal walls have no bulging or lesions, cervix pink with no lesions, scant clear mucoid discharge.
Bimanual: No pain on moving cervix, uterus anteflexed and anteverted, no enlargement or irregularity.
Adnexa: Ovaries not enlarged.
Rectal: No hemorrhoids, fissures, or lesions; no masses or tenderness; stool brown with FIT test negative.

ASSESSMENT

Genital structures intact and appear healthy

CHAPTER 19

Anus, Rectum, and Prostate

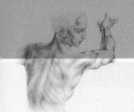

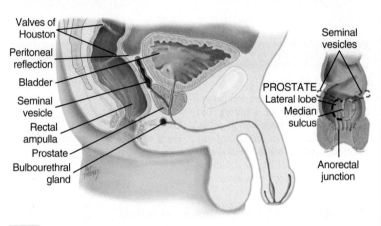

Valves of Houston
Peritoneal reflection
Bladder
Seminal vesicle
Rectal ampulla
Prostate
Bulbourethral gland

Seminal vesicles
PROSTATE
Lateral lobe
Median sulcus
Anorectal junction

19.1 The anal canal, rectum, and male prostate.

The **anal canal** is the outlet of the gastrointestinal (GI) tract and is about 3.8 cm long in adults (Fig. 19.1). It slants forward toward the umbilicus, forming a distinct right angle with the rectum, which rests back in the hollow of the sacrum.

The anal canal is surrounded by two concentric layers of muscle: the *internal* and *external sphincters.*

The **rectum,** which is 12 cm long, is the distal portion of the large intestine. Just above the anal canal, the rectum dilates and turns posteriorly, forming the rectal ampulla.

In males the **prostate gland** lies in front of the anterior wall of the rectum. It surrounds the bladder neck and the urethra, and it secretes a thin, milky alkaline fluid that helps sperm viability. It has two lobes that are separated by a shallow groove called the **median sulcus**. The two **seminal vesicles** project like rabbit ears above the prostate. They secrete a fluid containing fructose, which nourishes the sperm.

SUBJECTIVE DATA

1. Usual bowel routine: frequency, stool color
2. Change in bowel habits: diarrhea, constipation, use of enemas
3. Rectal bleeding, blood in the stool
4. Medications: laxatives, stool softeners, iron
5. Rectal conditions (pruritus, hemorrhoids, fissure, fistula)
6. Family history: colon, rectal, prostate cancer; polyps; inflammatory bowel disease
7. Diet of high-fiber foods
8. Patient-centered care: HPV vaccine, stool blood test, colonoscopy, talk of prostate-specific antigen (PSA) blood test (for men)

OBJECTIVE DATA

PREPARATION

Examine the male in the left lateral decubitus position or standing and leaning over an examination table. Place the female in the lithotomy position if examining the genital area as well; use the left lateral decubitus position for the rectal area alone.

EQUIPMENT NEEDED

Penlight
Lubricating jelly
Glove
Fecal occult blood test materials

Normal Range of Findings	Abnormal Findings
Inspect the Perianal Area	
The anus normally appears moist and hairless, with coarse, folded, pigmented skin. The anal opening is tightly closed. There are no lesions.	Inflammation. Lesions or scars. Linear split—Fissure. Flabby skin sac—Hemorrhoid. Shiny blue skin sac—Thrombosed hemorrhoid. Small round opening in anal area—Fistula.
The sacrococcygeal area appears smooth and even.	Inflammation or tenderness, swelling, a tuft of hair, or a dimple at the tip of the coccyx may indicate pilonidal cyst (see Table 19.1, Abnormalities of the Anal Region, p. 263).
Instruct the person to hold his or her breath and bear down by performing a Valsalva maneuver. There should be no break in skin integrity or protrusion through the anal opening.	Appearance of fissure or hemorrhoids. Circular red doughnut of tissue— Rectal prolapse.

Normal Range of Findings	Abnormal Findings

Palpate the Anus and Rectum

Drop lubricating jelly onto your gloved index finger. Inform the person that palpation is not painful but it may feel as if he or she needs to move the bowels.

Place the pad of your index finger gently against the anal verge. You will feel the sphincter tighten and then relax (Fig. 19.2). As it relaxes, flex the tip of your finger and slowly insert it into the anal canal in a direction toward the umbilicus.

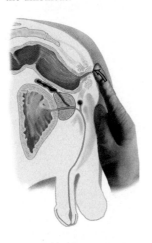

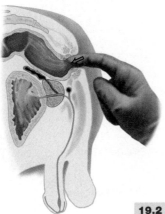

19.2

Normal Range of Findings	Abnormal Findings
Rotate your examining finger to palpate the entire muscular ring. The canal should feel smooth and even. To assess tone, ask the person to tighten the muscle. The sphincter should tighten evenly around your finger with no pain to the person.	Decreased tone. Increased tone occurs with inflammation and anxiety.
Above the anal canal the rectum turns posteriorly, following the curve of the coccyx and sacrum. Insert your finger farther and explore all around the rectal wall. It normally feels smooth with no nodularity. Promptly report any mass you discover for further examination.	Thrombosed internal hemorrhoid. A soft, slightly movable mass may be a polyp. A firm or hard mass with irregular shape or rolled edges may signify carcinoma (see Table 26.2, p. 726, in Jarvis: *Physical Examination and Health Assessment,* 8th ed.).

Palpate the Prostate Gland

In males palpate the prostate gland on the anterior wall (Fig. 19.3). Carefully press *into* the gland at each location.

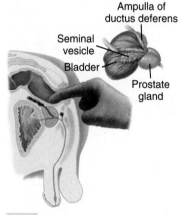

Ampulla of
ductus deferens

Seminal
vesicle

Bladder

Prostate
gland

19.3   Palpate the prostate gland.

NOTE:
- Size—2.5 cm long × 4 cm wide; should not protrude more than 1 cm into the rectum
- Shape—Heart shaped, with palpable central groove

Enlarged or atrophied gland.

Flat with no groove.

Normal Range of Findings	Abnormal Findings
• Surface—Smooth • Consistency—Elastic, rubbery • Mobility—Slightly movable • Sensitivity—Nontender to palpation	Nodular. Hard; or boggy, soft, fluctuant. Fixed. Tender. Enlarged, firm, smooth gland with obliterated central groove suggests benign prostatic hypertrophy (BPH). Swollen, exquisitely tender gland accompanies prostatitis. Any stone-hard, irregular, fixed nodule indicates carcinoma (see Table 26.3, p. 727, in Jarvis: *Physical Examination and Health Assessment,* 8th ed.).
Withdraw your examining finger; normally there is no bright red blood or mucus on the glove. Offer the person tissues to remove the lubricant and help him or her to a more comfortable position.	
Examination of Stool. Inspect any feces remaining on the glove. Normally the color is brown, and the consistency is soft.	Jellylike mucus shreds mixed in stool indicate inflammation. Bright red blood on stool surface indicates rectal bleeding. Bright red blood mixed with feces indicates possible colonic bleeding.
Test any stool on the glove for *occult* (or hidden) *blood.* Use the fecal immunochemical test (FIT) to detect small quantities of blood. A negative response is normal. If the stool is *positive,* it indicates occult blood. The FIT can be used without the diet or medication restrictions of the older guaiac-based tests. There are two types of FITs: liquid-based, which stores the stool sample in a hemoglobin-stabilizing buffer, and dry-slide cards, which are analyzed manually (Robertson et al., 2017).	Black, tarry stool with distinct malodor indicates upper gastrointestinal bleeding with blood partially digested. Black stool also occurs with ingesting iron medications or bismuth preparations. Gray, tan stool occurs with absent bile pigment, e.g., obstructive jaundice. Pale yellow, greasy stool occurs with increased fat content (steatorrhea), as occurs with malabsorption syndrome. Occult bleeding usually indicates cancer of colon.

Summary Checklist: Anus, Rectum, and Prostate Examination

1. **Inspect anus** and perianal area.
2. Inspect during Valsalva maneuver.
3. **Palpate anal canal** and rectum on all adults.
4. **Test stool** for occult blood.

You have asked about the PSA blood test as a warning for prostate cancer. We have this discussion at age 50 years for men who are at average risk of prostate cancer; at age 45 years for African-American men and for men who have a father, brother, or son diagnosed with prostate cancer at an early age (younger than 65 years); and at age 40 years for men at even higher risk, that is, men with more than one first-degree relative with prostate cancer at an early age (ACS, 2017a). We follow the test once a year and look for a sustained rise in the PSA level. A rising PSA does not mean it is cancer for sure; it means the gland is active, which occurs also with noncancerous growth, infection such as prostatitis, and ejaculation. The rising PSA can lead to further testing, such as radiologic imaging and a needle biopsy. These tests can be expensive (depending on health insurance), slightly painful, and can lead to worry while you wait for results. With PSA screening, 5-, 10-, and 15-year survival rates are close to 100%, 98%, and 94%, respectively (Peisch et al., 2017). It is not yet clear whether early detection and treatment of the slow-growing type of prostate cancer leads to any change in the natural history and outcome of the disease. Please discuss these points with your loved ones, and let us know whether to follow your PSA blood test.

Screening for colorectal cancer starts at age 50 years, and a colonoscopy is recommended for men and women. Colorectal cancer can be detected at a curable stage in people who have no warning symptoms. We have many good clinical trials showing lower death rates among people who have screening colonoscopy compared with those who do not (Inadomi, 2017). The colonoscopy also can show precancerous polyps, and these are removed during the test, which further decreases the risk of colorectal cancer. If the first colonoscopy shows no cancer and no polyps, the next test can be 10 years later.

DOCUMENTATION

Sample Charting

SUBJECTIVE

Has one BM daily, soft, brown, no pain, no change in bowel routine. On no medications. Has no history of pruritus, hemorrhoids, fissure, or fistula. Diet includes 1 to 2 servings daily each of fresh fruits and vegetables but no whole-grain cereals or breads.

OBJECTIVE

No fissure, hemorrhoids, fistula, or skin lesions in perianal area. Sphincter tone good, no prolapse. Rectal walls smooth, no masses or tenderness. Prostate not enlarged, no masses or tenderness. Stool brown, Hematest negative.

ASSESSMENT

Rectal structures intact, no palpable lesions

ABNORMAL FINDINGS

TABLE 19.1	Abnormalities of the Anal Region

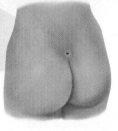
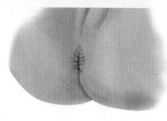

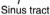
Sinus tract

Pilonidal Cyst or Sinus

A hair-containing cyst or sinus located in the midline over the coccyx or lower sacrum. Often opens as a dimple with visible tuft of hair and possibly an erythematous halo or may appear as a palpable cyst. When advanced, has a palpable sinus tract. Although it is a congenital disorder, the lesion is first diagnosed between the ages of 15 and 30 years.

Pruritis Ani

Intense itching and burning in the perineum has myriad causes: soaps, restrictive clothing, fecal soiling or hemorrhoids, eczema or psoriasis, STIs (herpes, condylomata), candida infection from moist or sweaty folds of obese or aging persons, many systemic causes (diabetes, liver disease), and pinworm infestation in children. Persistent scratching makes an inflammatory response and shows as red, raised, thickened, excoriated skin; may be swollen and moist. Careful history leads to treating the underlying cause. Urge person not to scratch and to avoid scented soap, prepared wipes, tight underclothing (Ansari, 2016; Swamiappan, 2016).

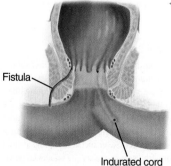

Fistula

Indurated cord

◀ Anorectal Fistula

Anorectal abscess starts from an infected anorectal gland; the infection channels through the perianal tissues to form a fistula, a connection between the infected gland and the outside perineum (Foxx-Orenstein, Umar, & Crowell, 2014). Fistulae also occur with Crohn disease or radiation therapy. Persistent pain and swelling occur with abscesses; fistulae are sometimes painful and itch. The fistula track feels like an indurated cord on bidigital palpation; it may drain purulent or serosanguineous matter.

Continued

| TABLE 19.1 | Abnormalities of the Anal Region—cont'd |

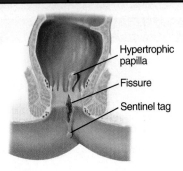

Hypertrophic papilla

Fissure

Sentinel tag

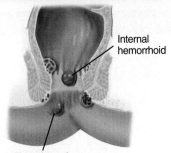

Internal hemorrhoid

Thrombosed external hemorrhoid

Fissure

An exquisitely painful longitudinal tear in the superficial mucosa at the anal margin. Most (>90%) occur in the posterior midline area. Pain is like passing "shards of glass"; may have bright red blood in the stool. An acute fissure has sharp edges, and a chronic fissure is indurated and accompanied by a papule of skin, *sentinel tag*, on the anal margin below or a polyp above. Fissures are caused by trauma, ischemia, and elevated anal pressure. Occurs with constipation, obesity, and hypothyroidism (Mapel, Schum, & Von Worley, 2014). Treatment medically is stool softeners, nitroglycerin ointment, or topical nifedipine or diltiazem cream, but injection of botulinum toxin into internal and anal sphincter is slightly more effective (Foxx-Orenstein, Umar, & Cromwell, 2014).

Hemorrhoids

These common flabby papules are due to a varicosed vein. An *external hemorrhoid* originates below the anorectal junction covered by anal skin. When *thrombosed,* it contains clotted blood and is a painful, swollen, shiny blue mass that itches and bleeds with defecation. When resolved, it leaves a painless, flabby skin sac around the anal orifice. An *internal hemorrhoid* is covered by mucous membrane. Hemorrhoids result from increased pressure: straining at stool, chronic constipation, pregnancy, obesity, low-fiber diet. Accompanied by painless rectal bleeding, red blood on tissue or toilet bowl, pruritus, anal swelling and pain, fecal soilage, mucus discharge. Treat with fiber supplement, laxative, decreased time on commode, rubber band ligation (Foxx-Orenstein, Umar, & Cromwell, 2014; Jacobs, 2014).

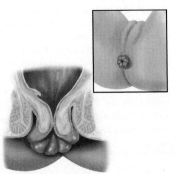

Rectal Prolapse

The complete rectal mucous membrane protrudes through the anus, appearing as a moist red doughnut with radiating lines. When prolapse is incomplete, only the mucosa bulges. When complete, it includes the anal sphincters. Occurs following a Valsalva maneuver such as straining at stool or with exercise. Caused by weakened pelvic support muscles and requires surgery.

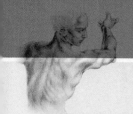

CHAPTER 20

The Complete Health Assessment

The following examination sequence combines all the separate steps into a complete and smoothly flowing assessment. The sequence puts steps in clusters by body region and proceeds systematically head to toe, concluding with examination of the genitalia. This is the most efficient way of conducting the examination, and it minimizes the number of position changes for you and the patient, thus avoiding tiring the patient. The running second column presents a sample recording when findings are within the normal and healthy range.

Sequence

The patient walks into the room and sits; the examiner sits facing the patient; the patient remains in street clothes.

Sample Recording

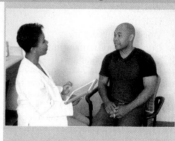

The Health History

1. Collect the history, complete or limited as visit warrants. While obtaining the history and throughout the examination, note data on the person's general appearance.

Sequence	Sample Recording

General Appearance

1. Appears stated age
2. Level of consciousness
3. Skin color
4. Nutritional status
5. Posture and position comfortably erect
6. Obvious physical deformities
7. Mobility:
   Gait
   Use of assistive devices
   Range of motion of joints
   No involuntary movement
8. Facial expression
9. Mood and affect
10. Speech:
    Articulation
    Pattern
    Content appropriate
    Native language
11. Hearing
12. Personal hygiene

The following lined rules indicate position change for examiner or patient.

(Patient's name) is a (age)-year-old (male/female), well nourished, well developed, who appears stated age. He is alert, oriented, cooperative, with no signs of acute distress. Appearance, behavior, and speech are appropriate; recent and remote memory intact.

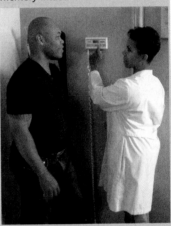

Measurement

1. Weight
2. Height
3. Waist circumference
4. Compute body mass index (BMI)
5. Vision using Snellen eye chart

Weight 78 kg (172 lbs), height 175 cm (5′9″), waist 35 inches, BMI 25, vision right eye 20/20, left eye 20/30—1.

Ask the patient to empty the bladder (save specimen if needed), to disrobe except for underwear, and to put on a gown. The patient sits with the legs dangling off the side of the bed or table; examiner stands in front of the person.

Skin

1. Examine both hands and inspect the nails.
2. For the rest of the examination, examine skin with corresponding regional examination.

Skin: Color light brown (tan-pink, brown, brown-black), warm to touch; turgor good, no lesions.
Nails: No clubbing or deformities, nail beds pink with prompt capillary refill.

Sequence	Sample Recording

Vital Signs

1. Radial pulse
2. Respirations
3. Blood pressure (BP)
4. Temperature
5. Pain assessment

TPR: 37°C–76–14, BP 128/ 84 mm Hg right arm, sitting. Denies pain.

Head and Face

1. Inspect and palpate scalp, hair, and cranium.
2. Inspect face: expression, symmetry (cranial nerve VII).
3. Palpate the temporal artery, then the temporomandibular joint as the person opens and closes the mouth.
4. Palpate the maxillary sinuses and frontal sinuses.

Hair: Head shaved. Head: Normocephalic, no lumps, no lesions, no tenderness. Face: Symmetric, no weakness, no involuntary movements.

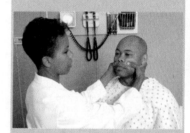

Eyes

1. Test visual fields by confrontation (cranial nerve II).
2. Test extraocular muscles: corneal light reflex, six cardinal positions of gaze (cranial nerves III, IV, VI).
3. Inspect external eye structures.
4. Inspect conjunctivae, sclerae, corneae, irides.
5. Test pupils: size, response to light, and accommodation (CN II, CN III).

Darken Room.

6. Using an ophthalmoscope inspect ocular fundus: red reflex, disc, vessels, and retinal background.

Eyes: Visual fields intact by confrontation. EOMs intact. Brows and lashes present. No ptosis. Conjunctivae clear. Sclerae white, no lesions. PERRLA. Fundi: Red reflex present bilaterally. Discs flat with sharp margins. Vessels present in all quadrants without crossing defects. Retinal background has even color with no hemorrhages or exudates. Macula has even color.

Sequence	Sample Recording
Ears	
1. Inspect external ear: position and alignment, skin condition, and auditory meatus.	*Ears: No masses, lesions, tenderness, or discharge. Both TMs pearly gray with light reflex and landmarks intact, no perforations. Whispered words heard bilaterally.*
2. Move auricle and push tragus for tenderness.	
3. Using an otoscope inspect the canal and then the tympanic membrane for color, position, landmarks, and integrity.	
4. Test hearing: whispered voice test.	
Nose	
1. Inspect external nose: symmetry, lesions.	*Nose: No deformity. Nares patent. Mucosa pink; no septal deviation or perforation.*
2. Test the patency of each nostril.	
3. Using a nasal speculum inspect the nares: nasal mucosa, septum, and turbinates.	
Mouth and Throat	
1. Using a penlight inspect the mouth: buccal mucosa, teeth and gums, tongue, floor of mouth, palate, and uvula.	*Mouth: Can clench teeth. Mucosa and gingivae pink; no masses or lesions. Teeth in good repair. Tongue protrudes in midline; no tremor.*
2. Grade tonsils if present.	*Throat: Mucosa pink, no lesions. Uvula arises in midline on phonation. Tonsils surgically absent. Gag reflex present.*
3. Note mobility of uvula as the person phonates "ahh" and test gag reflex (cranial nerves IX, X).	
4. Ask the person to stick out the tongue (cranial nerve XII).	
5. Palpate the mouth bimanually if indicated.	
Neck	
1. Inspect neck: symmetry, lumps, and pulsations.	*Neck: Supple with full ROM, no pain. Symmetric, no lymphadenopathy or masses; trachea midline; thyroid not palpable, no bruits. Carotid pulses 2+ and = bilaterally.*
2. Palpate the cervical lymph nodes.	
3. Inspect and palpate carotid pulse, one side at a time. If indicated, listen for carotid bruits.	

Sequence	Sample Recording

4. Palpate the trachea in midline.
5. Test range of motion (ROM) and muscle strength against your resistance: head forward and back, head turned to each side, and shoulder shrug (cranial nerve XI).

Step behind the person, taking your stethoscope.
6. Palpate thyroid gland.
Open the person's gown to expose all of the back but leave gown on shoulders and anterior chest.

Chest, Posterior and Lateral

1. Inspect the posterior chest: configuration of the thoracic cage, skin characteristics, and symmetry of shoulders and muscles.
2. Palpate: symmetric expansion, tactile fremitus, lumps, or tenderness.
3. Palpate length of spinous processes.
4. Percuss over all lung fields.
5. Percuss costovertebral angle, noting tenderness.
6. Auscultate breath sounds and note adventitious sounds.

Move around to face the patient; the patient remains sitting. At the time for the female breast examination, ask the woman's permission to lift the gown to drape on the shoulders, exposing the anterior chest; for a male, lower the gown to the lap.

Anterior Chest

1. Inspect: respirations and skin characteristics.
2. Palpate: tactile fremitus, lumps, and tenderness.
3. Percuss lung fields.
4. Auscultate breath sounds.

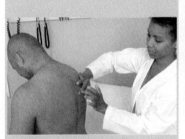

Chest: AP < transverse diameter. Respirations 16 per minute, relaxed and even. Chest expansion symmetric. Tactile fremitus equal bilaterally. Resonant to percussion over lung fields. Breath sounds clear. No adventitious sounds.

Sequence	Sample Recording

Heart

1. Ask the person to lean forward slightly and exhale briefly; auscultate base of the heart for any murmurs.

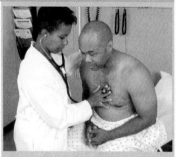

(See sample recording in HEART section on p. 271.)

Upper Extremities

1. Test range of motion and muscle strength of hands, arms, and shoulders.
2. Palpate the epitrochlear nodes.

(See sample recording in LOWER EXTREMITIES section on p. 272.)

Female Breasts

1. Inspect for symmetry, mobility, and dimpling as the woman lifts arms over the head, puts the hands on the hips, and leans forward.
2. Inspect supraclavicular and infraclavicular areas.

Breasts symmetric. No retraction, no nipple discharge, no lesions. Contour and consistency firm and homogeneous. No masses or tenderness. No lymphadenopathy.

Help the patient to lie supine with the head at a 30- to 45-degree angle. Stand at the person's right side. Drape the gown up across shoulders and place an extra sheet across the lower abdomen.

3. Palpate each breast, lifting the same side arm up over head. Include the tail of Spence and areola.
4. Palpate each nipple for discharge.
5. Support the person's arm and palpate the axilla and regional lymph nodes.
6. Teach breast self-examination.

Sequence	Sample Recording

Male Breasts

1. Inspect while palpating the anterior chest wall.
2. Supporting each arm, palpate the axilla and regional nodes.

Neck Vessels

1. Inspect each side of neck for a jugular venous pulse, turning the person's head slightly to the other side.
2. Estimate the jugular venous pressure if indicated.

External jugular veins flat.

Heart

1. Inspect precordium for pulsations and heave (lift).
2. Palpate the apical impulse and note the location.
3. Palpate the precordium for thrills.
4. Auscultate the apical rate and rhythm.
5. Auscultate with the diaphragm of the stethoscope to study heart sounds, inching from the apex up to the base or vice versa.
6. Auscultate the heart sounds with the bell of the stethoscope, again inching through all locations.
7. Turn the person over to the left side while again auscultating the apex with the bell.

Precordium: Apical impulse at 5th intercostal space, left midclavicular line. No heave or thrill; rate 68 per minute and rhythm regular; S_1 and S_2 are normal, not diminished or accentuated, no extra sounds, no murmurs.

The person should be supine, with the bed or table flat; arrange drapes to expose the abdomen from the chest to the pubis.

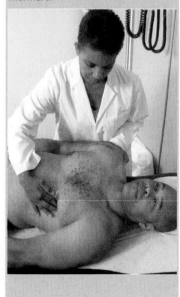

Sequence	Sample Recording

Abdomen

1. Inspect: contour, symmetry, skin characteristics, umbilicus, and pulsations.
2. Auscultate bowel sounds.
3. Auscultate for vascular sounds over the aorta and renal arteries.
4. Percuss all quadrants.
5. Palpate: light palpation in all quadrants, then deep palpation in all quadrants.
6. Palpate for liver, spleen, kidneys, and for aorta pulsation.
7. Test the abdominal reflexes if indicated.

Abdomen: Flat, symmetric with no apparent masses. Skin smooth with no striae, scars, or lesions. Bowel sounds present, no bruits. Tympany to percussion in all 4 quadrants. Abdomen soft to palpation, no organomegaly, no masses, no tenderness.

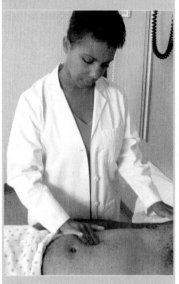

Inguinal Area

1. Palpate each groin for the femoral pulse and inguinal nodes.

Lift the drape to expose the legs.

Lower Extremities

1. Inspect: symmetry, skin characteristics, and hair distribution.
2. Palpate pulses: popliteal, posterior tibial, and dorsalis pedis.
3. Palpate for temperature and pretibial edema.
4. Separate toes and inspect.
5. Test range of motion and muscle strength: hips, knees, ankles, and feet.

Ask the patient to sit up and dangle the legs off the bed or table. Keep the gown on and drape it over the lap.

Extremities brown (pink-tan, brown-black) color with no redness, cyanosis, or skin lesions. Extremity size symmetric with no swelling or atrophy. Temperature warm and = bilaterally. All pulses present, 2+ and = bilaterally. No lymphadenopathy.

(See MUSCULOSKELETAL section on p. 274 for muscle sample recording.)

Sequence	Sample Recording

Musculoskeletal

1. Note muscle strength as person sits up.

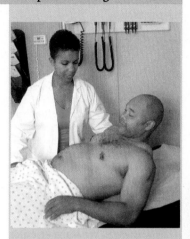

Neurologic

NOTE: Testing of cranial nerves II to XII was integrated during head and neck regional examinations.

1. Test sensation in selected areas on face, arms, hands, legs, and feet: superficial pain, light touch, and vibration.
2. Test position sense.
3. Test stereognosis.
4. Test cerebellar function of the upper extremities using finger-to-nose test or rapid alternating movements test.
5. Test the cerebellar function of the lower extremities by asking the person to run each heel down the opposite shin.
6. Elicit deep tendon reflexes (DTRs): biceps, triceps, brachioradialis, patellar, and Achilles.
7. Test the Babinski reflex.

Neurologic, sensory: Pinprick, light touch, vibration intact. Stereognosis—able to identify key.

Motor: No atrophy, weakness, or tremors. Rapid alternating movements (RAMs)—finger-to-nose smoothly intact.

Reflexes: Normal abdominal, DTRs all 2+ and equal bilaterally, no Babinski sign.

Ask the patient to stand with the gown on. Stand close to the patient.

Lower Extremities

1. Inspect lower legs for varicose veins.

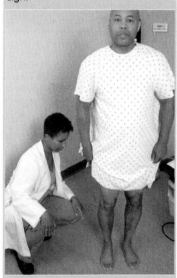

Sequence	Sample Recording
Musculoskeletal	

Musculoskeletal

1. Ask the person to walk across the room, turn, and walk back toward you in heel-to-toe fashion.
2. Ask the person to walk on the toes for a few steps and then to walk on the heels for a few steps.
3. Stand close and check the Romberg sign.
4. Ask the person to hold the edge of the bed and perform a shallow knee bend, one for each leg.
5. Stand behind and check the spine as the person touches the toes.
6. Stabilize the pelvis and test range of motion of the spine as the person hyperextends, rotates, and bends laterally.

Musculoskeletal: Gait smooth and fluid; able to tandem walk; negative Romberg sign. Joints and muscles symmetric; no swelling, masses, or deformity; normal spinal curvature. No tenderness to palpation of joints; no heat, swelling, or masses. Full ROM; movement smooth, no crepitance, no tenderness. Muscle strength—able to maintain flexion against resistance and without tenderness.

Sit on a stool in front of a male patient. The male stands.

Male Genitalia

1. Inspect the penis and scrotum.
2. Palpate the scrotal contents. If a mass exists, transilluminate.
3. Check for inguinal hernia.
4. Teach testicular self-examination.

Male genitalia: No lesions, no inflammation or discharge from penis. Scrotum—testes descended, symmetric; no masses. No inguinal hernia.

Ask an adult male to bend over the examination table, supporting the torso with his forearms on the table, and stand with the feet positioned with the toes turned inward. Help a bedfast male to a left lateral position with his right leg drawn up. The examiner stands.

Male Rectum

1. Inspect the perianal area.
2. With a gloved, lubricated finger, palpate the rectal walls and prostate gland.
3. Save a stool specimen for occult blood test.

Rectum: No fissures, hemorrhoids, fistulas, or skin lesions in perianal area. Sphincter tone good; no prolapse. Rectal walls smooth; no masses or tenderness. Prostate not enlarged; no masses or tenderness. Stool brown, hematest negative.

Help an adult female back to the examination table and help her into the lithotomy position. Drape her appropriately. Examiner sits on a stool at the foot of the table and then stands.

Sequence	Sample Recording
Female Genitalia	

1. Inspect the perineal and perianal areas.
2. Using a vaginal speculum, inspect the cervix and vaginal walls.
3. Procure specimens.
4. Perform a bimanual examination: cervix, uterus, and adnexa.
5. Continue the bimanual examination, checking the rectum and rectovaginal walls.
6. Save a stool specimen for occult blood test.
7. Help patient to a sitting position and provide tissues so she can wipe the perineal area.

External genitalia: No swelling, lesions, or discharge. No urethral swelling or discharge. *Internal genitalia:* Vaginal walls have no bulging or lesions; cervix pink with no lesions; scant clear mucoid discharge. *Bimanual:* No pain on moving cervix; uterus anteflexed and anteverted. *Adnexa:* Ovaries not enlarged.
Rectum: No hemorrhoids, fissures, or lesions; no masses or tenderness. Stool brown, hematest negative.

Tell the person that you are finished with the examination and that you will leave the room as he or she gets dressed. Return to discuss the examination and further plans and answer any questions. Thank the person for his or her time.

For the hospitalized patient, return the bed and any room equipment to the way you found it. Make sure the call light and telephone are within easy reach.

Recording the Data

Record the data from the history and physical examination as soon after the event as possible. Memory fades as your day progresses, especially when you are responsible for the care of more than one person.

It is difficult to strike a balance between recording too few data and recording too much data. It is important to remember that, from a legal perspective, if it is not documented, it was not done. Data important for the diagnosis and treatment of the person's health should be recorded, as well as data that contribute to your decision-making process. This includes charting relevant normal or negative findings.

On the other hand, a list of every assessment parameter yields an unwieldy, unworkable record. One way to keep your record complete yet succinct is to study your writing style. Use short, clear phrases. Avoid redundant introductory phrases such as, "The patient states that. ..." Avoid redundant descriptions such as, "no inguinal, femoral, or umbilical hernias." Just write, "no hernias."

Use simple line drawings to describe your findings. You do not need artistic talent; draw a simple sketch of a tympanic membrane, breast, abdomen, or cervix, and mark your findings on it. A clear picture is worth many sentences.

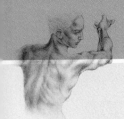

CHAPTER 21

Bedside Assessment and Electronic Documentation

In a hospital setting the patient does not require a complete head-to-toe physical examination during every 24-hour stay. The patient *does* require a consistent specialized exam at least every 12 hours that focuses on certain parameters. Note that some measurements such as daily weights, abdominal girth, or the circumference of a limb must be taken very carefully. The use of such measurements depends entirely on the consistency of the procedure from nurse to nurse.

Also remember that many assessments must be done frequently throughout the course of a shift. This chapter outlines the initial assessment that allows you to get to know your patient. As you perform this sequence, take note of anything that will need continuous monitoring such as an abnormal blood pressure or pulse oximetry reading or adventitious breath sounds. If there is no protocol in place for a particular assessment situation, decide for yourself how often you need to check on the person's status—it is very easy to be distracted by ringing bells and alarms as the shift progresses, but your own judgment about a patient's needs is just as important.

Sequence	Selected Photos
Wash your hands immediately upon entry to the room in front of the patient.	
Assist the person into bed. The patient is in bed with the bed at a comfortable level for the examiner.	

THE HEALTH HISTORY

On your way into the room, verify that any necessary markers or flags are in place at the doorway regarding such conditions as isolation precautions, latex allergies, or fall precautions. Once in the room, introduce yourself and let the patient know how long you will be the nurse.

Sequence	Selected Photos

Make direct eye contact and do not allow yourself to be distracted by intravenous (IV) pumps or other equipment as you ask how he or she is feeling and how he or she spent the previous shift.

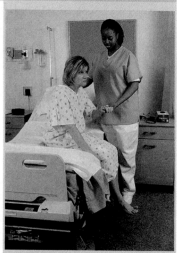

Assess for pain. "Are you currently having any pain or discomfort?" You should know when the last pain medication was given and what physician orders are written. Determine if further dosing is needed or if you need to contact the provider. Knowing the written orders, confirm settings on the patient-controlled analgesia (PCA) pump or epidural if in place. Confirm IV solution hanging matches orders for rate and type.

Offer water as a courtesy but also note the physical data that this gives you: the person's ability to hear, follow directions, cross the midline, and especially ability to swallow. As you collect this and subsequent history, note data on the general appearance listed in the following section. Verify that the correct name band has been applied to the wrist.

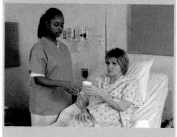

GENERAL APPEARANCE

1. Facial expression—Appropriate to the situation
2. Body position—Relaxed and comfortable or tense, in pain
3. Level of consciousness—Alert and oriented, attentive to your questions; responds appropriately
4. Skin color—Even tone consistent with racial heritage
5. Nutritional status—Weight appears in healthy range, even fat distribution, hydration appears healthy
6. Speech—Articulation clear and understandable, pattern fluent and even, content appropriate

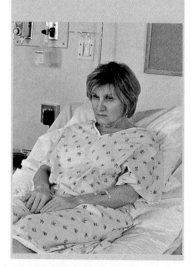

Sequence	Selected Photos

7. Hearing—Responses and facial expression consistent with what you have said
8. Personal hygiene—Ability to attend to basic hygiene such as brushing teeth and bathing

Measurement

1. Measure baseline vital signs (VS): temperature, pulse, respirations, BP. Note which arm to avoid for BP because of surgery, IV access. Collect and document VS more frequently if patient is unstable or patient condition changes. Know that VS are the ultimate responsibility of the nurse; the nursing assistant is not responsible for interpretation.

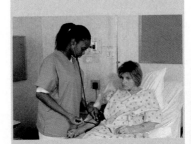

2. Pulse oximetry—Maintain ≥92% unless otherwise specified. Check pulse oximetry as ordered and as needed per nursing judgment. May need to monitor continuously if patient is lethargic, receiving oxygen, or receiving narcotics.
3. Ask patient to rate pain level on a 0-to-10 scale at this and every subsequent visit or VS measure. Note patient's ability to tolerate pain.
4. If pain medication is given, note response in 15 minutes for IV administration or 1 hour for oral dosing.

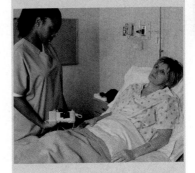

Sequence	Selected Photos

NEUROLOGIC SYSTEM

1. Eyes open spontaneously to name
2. Motor response is strong and equal bilaterally
3. Verbal responses make sense; speech is clear and articulate
4. Pupil size in mm and reaction, R and L
5. Muscle strength, R and L upper, using hand grips
6. Muscle strength, R and L lower, pushing feet against your palms
7. Any ptosis, facial droop
8. Sensation (omit unless indicated)
9. Communication
10. Ability to swallow

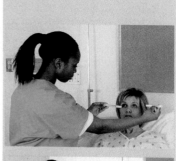

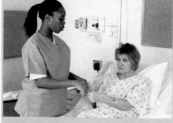

RESPIRATORY SYSTEM

1. Oxygen by mask, nasal cannula; check fitting and patient comfort
2. Note FIO_2
3. Respiratory effort
4. Auscultate breath sounds, comparing side to side:
   Posterior lobes: left upper, right upper, left lower, right lower
   NOTE: If not able to sit up, have patient roll, or ask for help to turn patient to the side
   Anterior lobes: right upper, left upper, right middle and lower, left lower
5. Cough and deep breathe; any mucus? Check color and amount.
6. Incentive spirometer if ordered; encourage patient to use every hour for 10 inspirations. If pulse oximetry % drops, encourage use every 15 minutes.

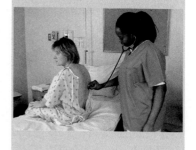

Sequence	Selected Photos

CARDIOVASCULAR SYSTEM

1. Auscultate rhythm at apex: regular, irregular? (Do NOT listen over gown.)
2. Check apical pulse against radial pulse, noting perfusion of all beats.
3. Assess heart sounds in all auscultatory areas: first with diaphragm; repeat with bell.
4. Check capillary refill for prompt return.
5. Check pretibial edema.
6. Palpate posterior tibial pulse, right and left.
7. Palpate dorsalis pedis pulse, right and left.

NOTE: Be prepared to assess pulses in the lower extremities by Doppler if you cannot find them by palpation.

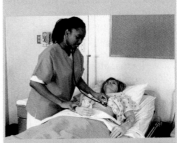
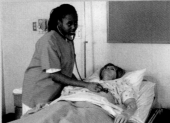
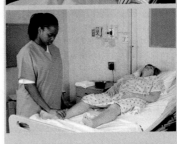

SKIN

1. Note skin color, consistent with person's racial heritage.
2. Palpate skin temperature; expect warm and dry.
3. Pinch a fold of skin under the clavicle or on the forearm to note mobility and turgor.
4. Note skin integrity, any lesions, and the condition of any dressings. Note any bleeding or infection, but do not change dressing until after physical exam.

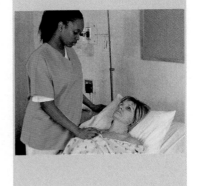

Sequence	Selected Photos

5. Assess IV site and note surrounding skin condition.
6. Complete any standardized scales used to quantify the risk of skin breakdown.
7. Verify that any air loss or pressure loss surfaces being used are applied properly and operating at the correct settings.

ABDOMEN

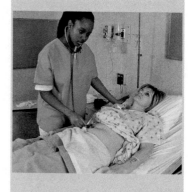

1. Assess contour of abdomen: flat, rounded, protuberant.
2. Listen to bowel sounds.
3. Check any drain for color and amount of drainage and insertion site integrity.
4. Inquire whether passing flatus or stool.
5. Knowing diet orders, determine if patient is tolerating ice chips, liquids, solids. Order correct diet as it is advanced. Note if patient is high risk for nutrition deficit.

GENITOURINARY

1. Inquire whether voiding regularly. Note: needs to void within 4 to 6 hours after surgery.
2. Check urine for color, clarity.
3. If Foley catheter is in place, check urine color, quantity, clarity with every VS check.
4. If urine output is below the expected value, perform a bladder scan according to agency protocol. Is the problem in the production of urine or its retention?

Sequence	Selected Photos

ACTIVITY

1. Knowing activity orders, if on bedrest, head of bed should be elevated. Is patient at high risk for skin breakdown?
2. Are sequential compression devices (SCDs) or thromboembolic deterrent (TED) hose in place? SCDs must be on patient 22 out of 24 hours to be effective.
3. If ambulatory, help patient sit and move to chair.
4. Note any assistance needed, how tolerates movement, distance walked to chair, ability to turn and sit.
5. Need for any ambulatory aid or equipment.
6. Complete any standardized scales used to quantify patient's risk for falling.
7. Initiate or continue appropriate Plan of Care. Check if any core measures apply, such as for heart failure. Implement core measures as appropriate.
8. Document assessment findings before leaving the room if possible.
9. Note exam findings requiring immediate attention:
- High or low BP (≤90 or ≥160 mm Hg systolic)
- High or low temperature (≤97° F or ≥100° F)
- High or low heart rate (≤60 or ≥95 bpm)
- High or low respirations (≤12 or ≥28/min)
- O₂ saturations ≤92%
- Low or no urine output (≤30 mL/hr or ≤240 mL/8 hr)
- Dark amber or bloody urine (except for urology patients)
- Postoperative nausea and/or vomiting
- Pain not controlled with medication

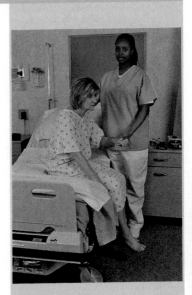

Sequence	Selected Photos

- Any unusual pain such as chest pain
- Bleeding
- Altered level of consciousness (LOC), confusion, or difficulty arousing
- Sudden restlessness and/or anxiety

ELECTRONIC CHARTING

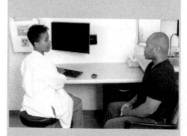

Most hospitals and clinics now use a basic or a comprehensive electronic health record (EHR) system. EHRs replace the paper medical record, placing all relevant patient information in an easily accessible electronic system. They do not include billing and scheduling systems but focus instead on patient information. One advantage of EHRs is the ability to access a lifetime of data to treat patients with chronic illness.

The meaningful use of EHRs, which include physician order entry and clinical decision support, may increase patient safety and quality care. EHRs allow all providers, regardless of geographic location, to access the health information, place orders, and receive timely patient status updates. No longer does a provider have to be on the clinical unit to retrieve test results, vital signs, or the most recent nurse's or physician's note.

Many health care organizations require providers to enter their own orders instead of allowing nurses to accept verbal or telephone orders. Computer provider order entry (CPOE) has decreased prescribing errors (Prgomet et al., 2016). Well-designed EHR systems can notify providers of potential medication interactions, dosage adjustments for renal patients or advanced age, and additional required testing (e.g., laboratory tests). Nurses can benefit from EHR use in medication administration through the use of bar-code scanners, which identify both the patient and the medication. Checklists built into EHR systems can help clinicians identify health care–associated infections or patients at risk for these infections. Checklists are also used for depression and suicide screening (Loudon, Nentin, & Silverman, 2016; Sudhanthar et al., 2015). Although no system is perfect, a well-designed EHR system can increase patient safety when successfully integrated into the workflow of a clinic or hospital. Unfortunately, EHRs are not always developed with the end user in mind, which can lead to issues with patient safety (Kellogg, Fairbanks, & Ratwani, 2017). As EHR use becomes the standard of care, more research is needed to determine the specific factors that contribute to patient safety and increased quality of care.

Using SBAR for Staff Communication

Throughout this text we have used the SOAP acronym (Subjective, Objective, Assessment, Plan) to organize assessment findings into written or charted communication. Now we turn to organizing assessment data for *verbal* communication (e.g., calls to providers, nursing shift reports, patient transfers to other units). For all these verbal reports, we use the SBAR framework: Situation, Background, Assessment, Recommendation.

SBAR is a standardized framework to transmit important, in-the-moment information. Using SBAR keeps your message concise and focused on the immediate problem yet gives your colleague enough information to grasp the current situation and make a decision. To formulate your verbal message, use these four points:

Situation. What is happening right now? Why are you calling? State your name, your unit, patient's name, room number, patient's problem, when it happened or when it started, how severe it is.

Background. Don't recite the patient's full history since admission. Do state the data pertinent to this moment's problem: admitting diagnosis, when admitted, and appropriate immediate assessment data, e.g., vital signs, pulse oximetry, change in mental status, allergies, current medications, IV fluids, lab results.

Assessment. What do YOU think is happening regarding the current problem? If you do not know, at least state which body system you think is involved. How severe is the problem?

Recommendation. What do you want the provider to do to improve the patient's situation? Here you offer probable solutions. Order more pain medication? Come and assess the patient?

Review the following examples of SBAR communication.

S: This is Bill on the Oncology Unit. I'm calling about Daniel Meyers in room 8417. He has refused all oral medications since 0800.

B: Daniel is a 59-year-old male with multiple myeloma. He was admitted for an autologous stem cell transplant and received chemotherapy 10 days ago. Now he is 5 days post auto transplant. Vital signs are stable. He is alert and oriented. IVs are dextrose 5% water running at 50 mL/hr. As of 1 hour ago he is feeling extreme nausea, refusing all food and oral meds.

A: I think the chemo he had pre-transplant is hitting him now. Nausea is getting worse despite Zofran.

R: I'm concerned that he cannot stay hydrated and he needs his meds. I need you to please change the IV rate and change all scheduled oral meds to IV. I also think we need to add an additional PRN antiemetic.

S: This is Andrea. I'm the nurse taking care of Max Goodson in 6443.

His condition has changed, and his most recent vital signs show a significant drop in blood pressure.

B: Max is 40 years old with a history of alcohol addiction. He was admitted through the ED last night with abdominal pain and a suspected GI bleed. His BPs have been running in the 130s/80s. He just had a large amount of liquid maroon stool and reported feeling dizzy. I rechecked his vitals; his BP is 88/50, and heart rate is 104.

A: I'm worried that his GI bleed is getting worse.

R: Will you order a STAT complete blood count and place an order to transfuse red blood cells if his hemoglobin is below 8 mg/dL? Also, can you please come and assess? I think we may need to drop an NG tube and lavage him.

Fig. 1.1 Adapted from the American Society of Human Genetics, www.ashg.org, 2004.

Fig. 4.1 Copyright Pat Thomas, 2010.

Table 5.3 Copyright Pat Thomas, 2010.

Table 5.4 Copyright Pat Thomas, 2010.

Table 5.5 From Potter, P. A., & Perry, A. G. (2009). *Fundamentals of nursing* (7th ed.). St. Louis: Mosby.

Fig. 7.1 Copyright © Pat Thomas, 2006.

Table 7.1 Copyright © Pat Thomas, 2010.

Table 7.2 Copyright © Pat Thomas, 2010.

Fig. 8.2 Copyright © Pat Thomas, 2010.

Table 8.1 (**Excessive cerumen and otitis externa**) Copyright © Pat Thomas, 2010; (**Retracted drum**) Adams, G. L., Bois, L. R., & Hilger, P. A. (1989). *Boies fundamentals of otolaryngology: A textbook of ear, nose, and throat diseases* (6th ed.). Philadelphia: Saunders; (**Otitis Media with Effusion [OME]**) Swartz, M. H. (2010). *Textbook of physical diagnosis: History and examination* (6th ed.). Philadelphia: Saunders; (**Acute purulent otitis media—early stage; Acute purulent otitis media—later stage**) Adams, G. L., Bois, L. R., & Hilger, P. A. (1989). *Boies fundamentals of otolaryngology: A textbook of ear, nose, and throat diseases* (6th ed.). Philadelphia: Saunders; (**Perforation**) Dhillon, R. S., & East, C. A. (2013). *Ear, nose and throat and head and neck surgery* (4th ed.). Philadelphia: Churchill Livingstone.

Figs. 9.1 and 9.2 Copyright © Pat Thomas, 2006.

Fig. 9.3 Copyright © Pat Thomas, 2010.

Table 9.1 (**Foreign body; Acute rhinitis; Allergic rhinitis**) Fireman, P. (1996). *Atlas of allergies* (2nd ed.). London: Mosby. (**Perforated septum**) Hawke, M. (1998). *Diagnostic handbook of otorhinolaryngology.* London: Martin Dunitz, reproduced by permission of Taylor & Francis Books UK.

Table 9.2 (**Cheilitis [angular stomatitis, perleche]**) Bolognia, J. L., Schaffer, J. V., Duncan, K. O., & Ko, C. J. (2014). *Dermatology essentials.* St. Louis: Elsevier. Courtesy of Louis A. Fragola, Jr., MD; (**Herpes simplex I**) Callen, J. P., Greer, K. E., Hood, A. F., et al. *Color atlas of dermatology,* Philadelphia, Saunders, 1993, p. 168; (**Gingivitis**) Newman, M. G., Takei, H. H., Klokkevold, P. R., et al. (2015). *Carranza's clinical periodontology* (12th ed.). St. Louis: Elsevier; (**Aphthous ulcers**) Sleisinger, M. H., & Fordtran, J. S. (1993). *Gastrointestinal diseases: Pathophysiology, diagnosis, and management* (5th ed.), vol. 1, Philadelphia: Saunders, Color plate WVII-B; (**Torus palatinus**) Courtesy Lemmi & Lemmi, 2011; (**Carcinoma**) Wenig B.M., Hefess C.S., & Adair, C.F. (1997). *Atlas of endocrine pathology,* Philadelphia: Saunders; (**Acute tonsillitis and pharyngitis**) Douglas, G., Nicol, F., & Robertson, C. (2013). *Macleod's clinical examination* (13th ed.). Philadelphia: Churchill Livingstone.

Figs. 10.1 and 10.2 Copyright © Pat Thomas, 2010.

Fig. 10.3 Copyright © Pat Thomas, 2014.

Fig. 10.7 Copyright © Pat Thomas, 2014.

Figs. 11.1 and 11.2 Copyright © Pat Thomas, 2010.

Fig. 12.2 Copyright © Pat Thomas, 2006.

Table 12.2 Copyright © Pat Thomas, 2006.

Figs. 13.1, 13.2, and 13.3 Copyright © Pat Thomas, 2010.

Figs. 14.1 and 14.2 Copyright © Pat Thomas, 2006.

Table 15.1 (**Ankylosing Spondylitis**) Copyright © Pat Thomas, 2018.

Fig. 15.2 Copyright © Pat Thomas, 2006.

Fig. 15.8 Courtesy Lemmi & Lemmi, 2011.

Figs. 16.1, 16.2, and 16.3 Copyright © Pat Thomas, 2006.

Fig. 16.19 Copyright © Pat Thomas, 2014.

Table 16.2 Copyright © Pat Thomas, 2006.

Fig. 17.1 Copyright © Pat Thomas, 2010.

Table 17.1 Copyright © Pat Thomas, 2006.

Aberger, M., Wilson, B., Holzbeierlein, J. M., et al. (2014). Testicular self-examination and testicular cancer: A cost-utility analysis. *Cancer Med*, 3(6), 1629–1634.

American Cancer Society (ACS). (2017a). *ACS recommendations for prostate cancer early detection*. https://www.cancer.org/cancer/prostate -cancer/early-detection/acs-recommendations .html.

American Cancer Society (ACS). (2017b). *Cancer facts & figures 2017*. https://www.cancer.org/ cancer-facts-and-figures-2017.pdf.

American Cancer Society. (2018). *Breast cancer facts & figures 2017-2018*. www.cancer.org.

American Heart Association. (2012). Measurement and interpretation of the ankle-brachial index. *Circulation*, 126(24), 2890–2909.

American Speech Language Hearing Association (ASHA). (2017). *Cleft lip and palate: Incidence and prevalence*. http://www.asha.org/PRP SpecificTopic.aspx?folderid=8589942918 &section=Incidence_and_Prevalence.

Ansari, P. (2016). Pruritus ani. *Clin Colon Rectal Surg*, 29(1), 38–42.

Benjamin, E. J., Blaha, M. J., Chiuve, S. E., et al. (2017). Heart disease and stroke statistics— 2017 Update: A report for the American Heart Association. *Circulation*, 135(10), e146–e603.

Berenson, A. B., Rahman, M., & Wilkinson, G. (2009). Racial difference in the correlates of bone mineral content/density and age at peak among reproductive-aged women. *Osteopor Int*, 20(8), 1439–1449.

Biro, F. M., Greenspan, L. C., Galvez, M. P., et al. (2013). Onset of breast development in a longitudinal cohort. *Pediatrics*, 132, 1019–1027.

Burns, C. E., Dunn, A. M., Brady, M. A., et al. (2013). *Pediatric primary care* (5th ed.). Philadelphia: Elsevier.

Carnethon, M. R., Jia, P., Howard, G., et al. (2017). Cardiovascular health in African Americans. *Circulation*, 136(21), e393–e423.

Carter, B. D., Abnet, C. C., & Feskanich, D. (2015). Smoking and mortality: Beyond established causes. *N Engl J Med*, 372(7), 631–640.

Centers for Disease Control and Prevention (CDC). (2017). *Most recent asthma data*. https://www. cdc.gov/asthma/most_recent_data.htm.

Chen, X., Stoner, J. A., Montgomery, P. S., et al. (2017). Prediction of 6-minute walk performance in patients with peripheral artery disease. *J Vasc Surg*, 2017(66), 1202–1209.

Criqui, M. H., & Aboyans, V. (2015). Epidemiology of peripheral artery disease. *Circ Res*, 116, 1509–1526.

Crocker, M. K., Stern, E. A., Sedaka, N. M., et al. (2014). Sexual dimorphisms in the associations of BMI and body fat with indices of pubertal development in girls and boys. *J Clin Endocrinol Metab*, 99, e1519–e1529.

Delmore, B. A., & Ayello, E. A. (2017). Pressure injuries caused by medical devices and other objects. *Am J Nurs*, 117(12), 36–46.

Foxx-Orenstein, A. E., Umar, S. B., & Crowell, M. D. (2014). Common anorectal disorders. *Gastro & Hepat*, 10(5), 294–301.

Gupta, D., & Chen, P. P. (2016). Glaucoma. *Am Fam Phys*, 93(8), 668–674.

Gutierrez, J., & Williams, O. A. (2014). A decade of racial and ethnic stroke disparities in the United States. *Neurology*, 82(12), 1080–1082.

Herman-Giddens, M. E., Slora, E. J., Wasserman, R. C., et al. (1997). Secondary sexual characteristics and menses in young girls seen in office practice. *Pediatrics*, 99(4), 505–512.

Herman-Giddens, M. E., Steffes, J., Harris, D., et al. (2012). Secondary sexual characteristics in boys. *Pediatrics*, 130(5), e1058–e1068.

Hollerbach, A. D., & Sneed, N. V. (1990). Accuracy of radial pulse assessment by length of counting interval. *Heart Lung*, 19(3), 258–264.

Hunter, D. J. (2015). Viscosupplementation for osteoarthritis of the knee. *N Engl J Med*, 372(11), 1040–1047.

Inadomi, J. M. (2017). Screening for colorectal neoplasia. *N Engl J Med*, 376(2), 149–156.

International Association for the Study of Pain. (2018). *Pain*. http://www.iasp-pain.org/index. aspx.

Islami, F., Sauer, A. G., Miller, K. D., et al. (2018). Proportion and number of cancer cases and deaths attributable to potentially modifiable risk factors in the United States. *CA: Cancer J Clin*, 68(1), 31–54.

Jacobs, D. (2014). Hemorrhoids. *New Engl J Med*, 371(10), 944–951.

Jamault, V., & Duff, E. (2013). Adolescent concussions: When to return to play. *Nurse Pract*, 38(2), 17–21.

Kaiser, P. K., Friedman, N. J., & Pineda, R. (2014). *The Massachusetts Eye and Ear Infirmary illustrated manual ophthalmology* (4th ed.). Philadelphia: Saunders.

Katz, A. (2017). Human papillomavirus-related oral cancers. *Am J Nurs*, 117(1), 34–40.

Khera, A. V., Emdin, C. A., Drake, I., et al. (2016). Genetic risk, adherence to a healthy lifestyle, and coronary disease. *N Engl J Med*, 375(24), 2349–2358.

Kellogg, K. M., Fairbanks, R. J., & Ratwani, R. M. (2017). EHR usability: Get it right from the start. *Biomed Instrument Tech*, 51, 197–199.

Kroenke, K., Spitzer, R. L., Williams, J. B. W., et al. (2007). Anxiety disorders in primary care: Prevalence, impairment, comorbidity, and detection. *Ann Intern Med*, 146, 317–325.

Lakkis, N. A., & Mahmassani, D. M. (2015). Screening instruments for depression in primary care: A concise review for clinicians. *Postgrad Med*, 127(1), 99–106.

Lin, S. N., Taylor, J., Alperstein, S., et al. (2014). Does speculum lubricant affect liquid-based Papanicolaou test adequacy? *Cancer Cytopathol*, 122(3), 221.

Loudon, H., Nentin, F., & Silverman, M. E. (2016). Using clinical decision support as a means of implementing a universal postpartum depression screening program. *Arch Womens Ment Health*, 19, 501–505.

Mapel, D. W., Schum, M., & Von Worley, A. (2014). The epidemiology and treatment of anal fissures in a population-based cohort. *BMC Gastroenterol*, 14(1), 129–135.

McGee, S. (2018). *Evidence-based physical diagnosis* (4th ed.). St. Louis: Elsevier.

Mochari-Greenberger, H., Xian, Y., Hellkamp, A. S., et al. (2015). Racial/ethnic and sex differences in emergency medical services transport among hospitalized US stroke patients. *J Am Heart Assoc*, 4(8), e002099.

Mozaffarian, D., Benjamin, E. J., Go, A. S., et al. (2016). Heart disease and stroke statistics—2016 update. *Circulation*, 133, e38–e360.

Mundy, K. M., Nichols, E., & Londsey, J. (2016). Socioeconomic disparities in cataract prevalence, characteristics, and management. *Semin Ophthalmol*, 3194, 358–363.

Nam, H. S., Kweon, S. S., Choi, J. S., et al. (2013). Racial/ethnic differences in bone mineral density among older women. *J Bone Mineral Metab*, 31(2), 190–198.

National Council on Aging (NCOA). *Take control of your health: 6 steps to prevent a fall*. https://www.ncoa.org/healthy-aging?falls-prevention.

National Institute of Neurological Disorders and Stroke (NINDS). (2017). *Brain basics: Preventing stroke*. https://www.ninds.nih.gov/Disorders/Patient-Caregiver-Education/Preventing-Stroke.

National Institutes of Health (NIH). (2014). *Dental caries (tooth decay) in children (age 2 to 11)*. https://www.nidcr.nih.gov/DataStatistics/FindDataByTopic/DentalCaries/DentalCariesChildren2to11.htm.

National Institutes of Health (NIH). (2017). *Your baby's hearing screening*. https://www.nided.nih.gov/health/your-babys-hearing-screening.

National Pressure Ulcer Advisory Panel (NPUAP). (2016). *NPUAP pressure injury stages*. http://www.npuap.org/resources/educational-and-clinical-resources/npuap-pressure-injury-stages/.

Nazare, J., Smith, J., Borel, A., et al. (2015). Usefulness of measuring both body mass index and waist circumference for the estimation of visceral adiposity and related cardiometabolic risk profile (from the INSPIRE ME IAA Study). *Am J Cardiol*, 115, 307–315.

Peisch, S. F., Van Blarigan, E. L., Chan, J. M., et al. (2017). Prostate cancer progression and mortality. *World J Urol*, 35(6), 867–874.

Preston, A., Rao, A., Strauss, R., et al. (2017). Deep tissue pressure injury. *Am J Nurs*, 117(5), 50–57.

Prgomet, M., Li, L., Niazkhani, Z., et al. (2016). Impact of commercial computerized provider order entry (CPOE) and clinical decision support systems (CDSSs) on medication errors, length of stay, and mortality in intensive care units: A systematic review and meta-analysis. *J Am Med Inform Assoc*, 24, 413–422.

Prokop-Prigge, K. A., Thaler, E., Wysocki, C. J., et al. (2014). Identification of volatile organic compounds in human cerumen. *J Chromatogr B Analyt Technol Biomed Life Sci*, 953-954, 48–52.

Robertson, D. J., Lee, J. K., Boland, C. R., et al. (2017). Recommendations on fecal immunochemical testing to screen for colorectal neoplasia. *Gastroint Endosc*, 85(1), 2–21.

Rosa-Olivares, J., Porro, A., Rodriguez-Varela, M., et al. (2015). Otitis Media. *Pediatr Rev*, 36(11), 480–488.

Schmit, K. M., Wansaula, Z., Pratt, R., et al. (2017). Tuberculosis – United States, 2016. *MMWR*, 66, 289–294.

Sudhanthar, S., Thakur, K., Sigal, Y., et al. (2015). Improving validated depression screen among adolescent population in primary care practice using electronic health records (EHR). *BMJ Qual Improv Rep*, 21(4).

Swamiappan, M. (2016). Anogenital Pruritus. *J Clin Diag Res*, 10(4), 1–3.

Swanton, C., & Govindan, R. (2016). Clinical implications of genomic discoveries in lung cancer. *N Engl J Med*, 374(19), 1864–1873.

Taurog, J. D., Chhabra, A., & Colbert, A. A. (2016). Ankylosing spondylitis and axial spondyloarthritis. *N Engl J Med*, 374(26), 2563–2574.

Tawfik, K. O., Ishman, S. L., Altaye, M., et al. (2017). Pediatric acute otitis media in the era of pneumococcal vaccination. *Otolaryngol*, 156(5), 938–945.

Van Schayck, O. C. P., Williams, S., & Barchilon, V. (2017). Treating tobacco dependence: Guidance for primary care on life-saving interventions. *NPJ Prim Care Respir Med*, 27(38), 1–12.

Varma, R., Vajaranant, T., Burkemper, B., et al. (2016). Visual impairment and blindness in adults in the United States from 2015 to 2050. *JAMA Ophthalmol*, 134(7), 802–809.

Vaughan, A. S., Ritchey, M. D., Hannan, J., et al. (2017). Widespread recent increases in county-level heart disease mortality across age groups. *Ann Epidemiol*, 27, 796–800.

Wellbrock, C. (2016). Melanoma and the microenvironment: Age matters. *N Engl J Med*, 375(7), 696–698.

INDEX

Page numbers followed by *b* indicates boxed material, *f* indicates illustrations, and *t* indicates tables.